CRPS/RS
Facts, Fiction and

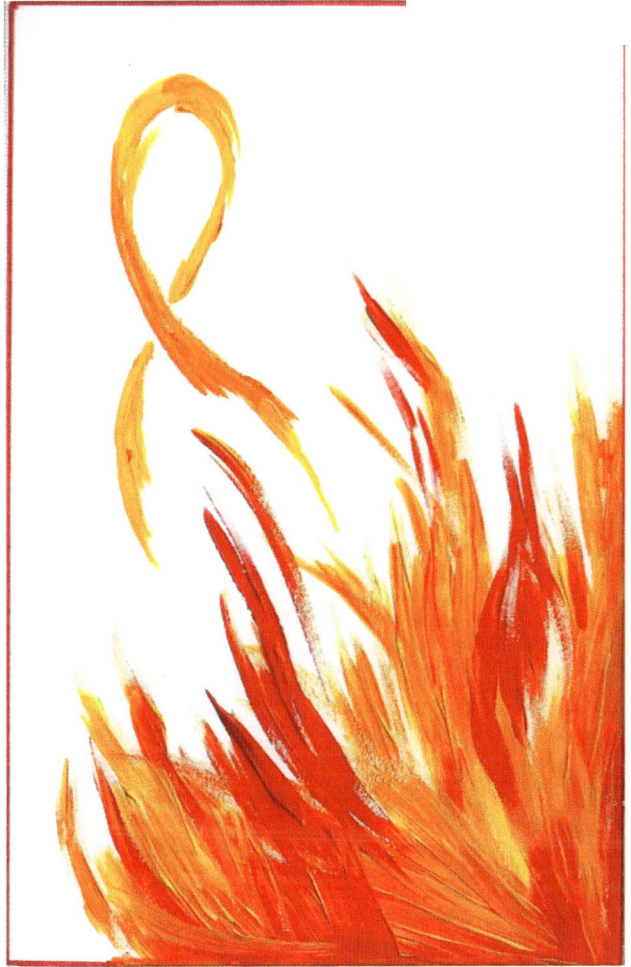

By
Nancy Renée Cotterman, RN
Preface by
Dr Pradeep Chopra , MD

ISBN:1494827344
ISBN-13: 9781494827342

DEDICATION

Dedicated to all those who have CRPS.

My Family for sticking with me when things got tough.

My friends who stuck with me when everyone else fled (The Adams, Tara Kochanek, and Amy Wallace.

A special thank you to my neighbor
Leonides Edwin Villalon MD who painted the artwork used on the cover.

A special thanks to Dr Pradeep Chopra, MD for his contribution and always being there when I need him.

Foreword

Pradeep Chopra, MD

Pain is one of the best protective mechanisms in our body. It protects and warns us against harm. In CRPS (Complex Regional Pain Syndrome) , pain becomes a disease by itself. It is no longer a protection but harmful to us. As a Pain Medicine specialist I have been treating and teaching the subject of chronic pain and especially CRPS for many years. I have read and continue to read all that there is on the subject. Which, brings me to the subject of Nancy Cotterman's book on CRPS. Books written by patients on CRPS are highly biased and clouded by their own personal experiences with the condition. I have been disappointed with the poor facts and low quality of work in the books written by people with CRPS that are currently available. This book fills a big need for high quality information for people with CRPS. This book is full of excellent information for people with CRPS and their caregivers, it is unbiased, factual and well illustrated. Nancy brings in a unique perspective both as a person with CRPS, a nurse and educator. As a physician, I find CRPS to be a challenge and it has become a passion with me to help as many people as I can. To understand the condition better I needed to talk to people who had dealt with CRPS and had tried different treatments. Nancy has been an immense source of knowledge, inspiration and a mentor to me in understanding CRPS.

Some of the best features of the book are that it is gives the reader the facts and experiences by real life examples of patients with CRPS. Nancy has used her extensive experience with her own condition and in helping hundreds of people around the country for the last 15 years to keep the book unbiased at the same time bringing to light the practical points in dealing with the condition. What I admire most about the book is that Nancy has gone to great lengths to keep the book unbiased and factual. She has tapped into her nursing education and her vast experience from helping people with CRPS for years. There are ample pictures to help the reader visualize some of the presentations of this condition. Pictures describe are a thousand words when it comes to making the reader understand things like skin color change, changes to muscles and nails. The book has gone in to great detail about treatment options – the good and the not so good. The book also addresses major issues as in dealing with finances, coping with the loss of function and learning to build a new life and moving forward. The stories in the book are real, about real people with CRPS. They are inspiring and factual.

I cannot help but talk to the reader about the author Nancy Renee Cotterman. She was diagnosed to have CRPS in 1996 after a car accident fractured her right foot. In 1996, little was known about CRPS. Over the years, Nancy raised a family of two beautiful daughters, one of whom is visually impaired. She is now proud grandmother. I have been very impressed with how Nancy has learnt to accept her condition, live a full life and also become a support to hundreds of other people around the world with CRPS. She is administrator of three Facebook support groups, CRPS mentor for ten years, has popular blog http://nancyCRPScrpsblog.blogspot.com, the director of a non profit organization (www.crpspartnersinpain.com) to raise funds for people with CRPS.

Nancy and I have strong passion to help people diagnosed with CRPS. Between the two us we cover most aspects about understanding CRPS. Medicine is an ever changing subject. As each day passes we learn more and more about management of CRPS. This book is an excellent treatise to use as a road map in your and our journey to living a full life despite CRPS.

Pradeep Chopra, MD
Assistant Professor (Clinical)
The Warren Alpert School of Brown Medicine,
Providence, RI
Director,
Pain Management Center.

CONTENTS

INTRODUCTION

INTRODUCTION

For most people, touch is the that we way express friendship and love. We shake hands as the socially accepted way to greet someone when we meet. A gentle caress tells someone that you love them, but for people with CRPS/CRPS even the slightest touch can bring excruciating pain to the recipient of that touch. CRPS/RSD causes the nervous system to go haywire. The nervous symptom perceives things like light touch as intense pain. While this condition is considered rare; it is more common than you might think. When it strikes someone, the person's entire life is affected. I know all too well how this disease can impact a person's life and the lives of the person's family and friends. I have Chronic Regional Pain Syndrome/Reflex Sympathetic Dystrophy (a.k.a. CRPS/RSD.)

The disease dates back to the Civil War. Some soldiers who were wounded would complain of extreme pain. They would describe it as if a fire were burning on the affected limb. Doctors recognized it as a disease but they didn't quite know how to treat it or why it developed in some soldiers and not others with the exact type of wound. In that era doctors didn't share theories or treatments with each other, each one worked with their own patients trying different things to try to reduce their patient's pain.

CRPS/RSD can be triggered by something as simple as a stubbed toe or a splinter, a sprain or a fracture, even medications such as Chemotherapy can be the cause. For me, it was a crushed foot that occurred when I was in a car accident. That was sixteen years ago. The past sixteen years have tested my strength, endurance and ability to cope. It has shown me who my real friends are and how much my family means to me. The purpose of this book is to help to medical professionals, care givers, family members and people with CRPS/RSD by providing information about the facts, fiction and feelings involved in CRPS/RSD. I have compiled a combination of medical information along with the emotions and feelings of those with CRPS/CRPS (from now on referred to as CRPS) and their caregivers.

This book will define CRPS/RSD. You will learn the importance of informed decision making with respect to the treatment of CRPS/RSD. Different treatment options will be explained including pros and cons of each treatment. You will be presented with the facts of CRPS and common misconceptions. The feelings that people with CRPS are faced with. Money is a big issue associated with CRPS. You will learn about Workman's Comp, Social Security Disability, and ADA compliance in the work place. Finally, you will read the stories of people with CRPS and their family members to see how CRPS affects no only the person who has it but their entire family.

CHAPTER 1
WHAT THE HECK IS CRPS/RSD?

I am a nurse. I can honestly say that we were never taught anything about CRPS/RSD in nursing school. Let's start with these initials. RSD stands for Reflex Sympathetic Dystrophy. It is also known as CRPS which stands for Complex Regional Pain Syndrome. It has also been known as causalgia. All of these names, are given to something that doctors and researchers don't completely understand. What we do know is that it is a chronic pain condition where an injury causes pain that is totally out of proportion for that injury and lasts long after the injury should have healed. We also know that CRPS affects the nerves, spinal cord and brain of the affected individual.

Today doctors and researchers still aren't one hundred percent clear on what causes CRPS to develop in one person and not in another with the same type of injury. Many physicians and nurses still do not know what CRPS is so they do not know how to diagnose and treat CRPS patients. There are many misconceptions about CRPS held within the medical community.

So what exactly is CRPS? It is a chronic neurological syndrome that is characterized by a severe burning pain that is often described by the people who have it as if someone poured lighter fluid on them and then lit them on fire. There are pathological changes in the bone and the skin, such as bone loss, and shinny, hairless reddish purple skin. Many people with CRPS have excessive sweating all of the time in the affective area(s). The tissues of the effective area(s) swell. Most have are extreme sensitivity to touch (allodynia).

Something as light as a breeze can cause excruciating pain. Clothing on the affecting area(s) can be painful. This last symptom can also cause people with CRPS to pull away from the ones that they love. Touch is a sign of friendship and love. Many people can't understand why you are constantly pushing them away and asking them not to touch you no matter how many times you explain why! Why? Because to someone with CRPS, touch is extremely painful.

Anyone can get CRPS It is more prevalent in women than men and there are an increasing number of cases in children being diagnosed. One of the biggest challenges that the CRPS patient face is the lack of proper understanding and education of pain management in the medical community. One of the biggest battles is that of getting treatments covered by health insurance and workman's compensation insurance. This can be both frustrating and cause a delay in treatment. Delay in treatment can also cause progression of the CRPS. Finally, the loss of employment, socialization and family life are all struggles that the person with CRPS may be faced with.

CRPS is a malfunction of part of the nervous system that usually develops in response to a traumatic even such as an accident or medical procedure. A minor injury such as a sprain, an IV stick, or a fall can all cause nerves to misfire sending constant pain signals to the brain. CRPS is broken down into two categories:

CRPS I (CRPS) – The symptoms of type I include: The presence of an initiating event such as a fracture, or sprain. Continuing pain including allodynia, which is pain from a normal stimulus, such as the breeze from a ceiling fan., Hyperalgesia which an increased sense of pain to an unpleasant stimuli. The pain is disproportionate to that associated with the injury. There is edema (swelling), changes in skin blood flow (skin color changes, skin temperature changes) and excessive sweating in the region of pain. For example: I have CRPS in my foot, a sheet touching my foot causes excruciating pain (allodynia). If someone accidentally stepped on my foot, the pain would be ten fold compared to someone stepping on the foot of someone without CRPS (hyperalgesia). The pain continues to feel as though the foot is still injured months and years after that injury had healed or the pain is more intense than it was at the time of the original injury.

The diagnosis of CRPS I (CRPS) is one of exclusion. It is based on the existence of conditions that would otherwise not account for the degree of pain and dysfunction. There is no one specific test or tests that can definitively diagnose CRPS, although some doctors do use several tests that will be described later as diagnostic tools; they are not definitive in diagnosing CRPS.

CRPS II (Causalgia) – In Type II, a definite nerve injury can be identified. The symptoms are the same as in type I, but the cause is different. This is the presence of constant pain, allodynia (pain resulting from normal stimulus) or hyperalgesia (an increased sense of pain) after an identifiable nerve injury. There is still evidence of edema, and skin changes. This diagnosis is also one of exclusion based on the existence of conditions that would otherwise account for the degree of pain and dysfunction from a nerve injury.

Cause of CRPS/RSD Current research suggest that the mechanism by which an injury triggers CRPS/RSD is unclear. The figure below is intended to give you a simplified view of how an injury might lead to the symptoms of CRPS/RSD

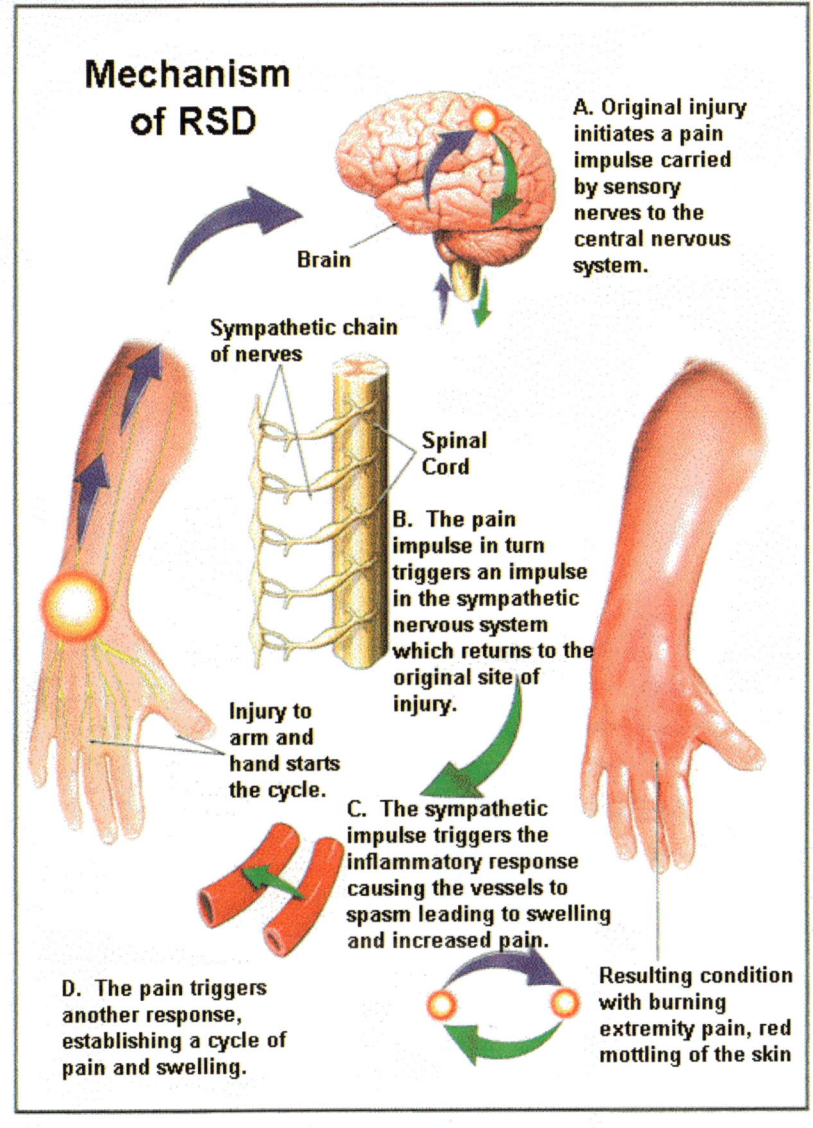

Mechanism of RSD

A. Original injury initiates a pain impulse carried by sensory nerves to the central nervous system.

Brain

Sympathetic chain of nerves

Spinal Cord

B. The pain impulse in turn triggers an impulse in the sympathetic nervous system which returns to the original site of injury.

Injury to arm and hand starts the cycle.

C. The sympathetic impulse triggers the inflammatory response causing the vessels to spasm leading to swelling and increased pain.

D. The pain triggers another response, establishing a cycle of pain and swelling.

Resulting condition with burning extremity pain, red mottling of the skin

Activation of the sympathetic nervous system following an injury is part of a fright–flight response to an emergency situation. This response is very important for survival. When we face an emergency situation the firing of sympathetic nerves causes blood vessels in the skin to contract, forcing blood deep into muscle. It enables us to use our muscle to get up after an acute injury and escape from further danger. Additionally the decreased supply of blood to the skin reduces blood loss through superficial injuries that may occur on the surface of the body. Ordinarily, the sympathetic nervous system shuts down within minutes to hours after an injury. For reasons we do not completely understand, individuals who go on to develop CRPS/ CRPS, the sympathetic nervous system appears to assume an abnormal function. Theoretically, this sympathetic activity at the site of injury could cause an inflammatory response causing the blood vesselsCRPS to spasm leading to more swelling and pain. (See B, C, and D in the figure above) The events could lead to more pain which triggers another response, establishing a vicious cycle of pain. The nerves then "memorize" these responses and cause changes within the nerves, spinal cord, and brain that become CRPS.

There are several new theoretical approaches involving the glial cell. A glial cell is defined as: a supportive cell in the central nervous system that unlike neurons, glial cells do not conduct electrical impulses. The glial cells surround neurons and provide support for and insulation between them. Glial cells are the most abundant cell types in the central nervous system. New studies regarding CRPS target the negative consequences of glial activation. Other theories being studied are that CRPS is caused by neuroinflammation and that it is an autoimmune disease. Researchers at the writing of this book are looking into these different possible causes that allow two people to have the same injury while one goes on to heal normally and the other to develop CRPS. By better understanding the changes that take place within the nervous system, we can develop better treatments for those with CRPS and better manage their symptoms.

CHAPTER 2
THE SYMPTOMS

CRPS often occurs after an injury or surgery to one of the limbs. The most prominent symptom of CRPS is pain. Other classic symptoms of RSD include: a change in color and temperature of the affected area, burning pain, changes in the nails, bones and muscles. While most people with RSD experience several of these symptoms, some experience them all. The affected area (an extremity, the back, the face, etc.) becomes a reddish purple in color. This color becomes more prominent when the person with RSD has a flare of their symptoms. The temperature of the affected area is cooler than the other parts of the body. Temperature probes that are extremely sensitive to the slightest changes in temperature can be used to check the temperature of the affected area compared to the unaffected areas. If your right foot has RSD, the temperature of different areas of that foot are taken and compared to the same areas of the unaffected foot. The affected foot will be cooler than the unaffected foot. Even without these instruments, you can feel the difference in temperature simply by touching to two feet. In addition to color and temperature changes in the skin; often the hair density changes as well. The skin becomes shinny. Below are some photos of what RSD can look like:

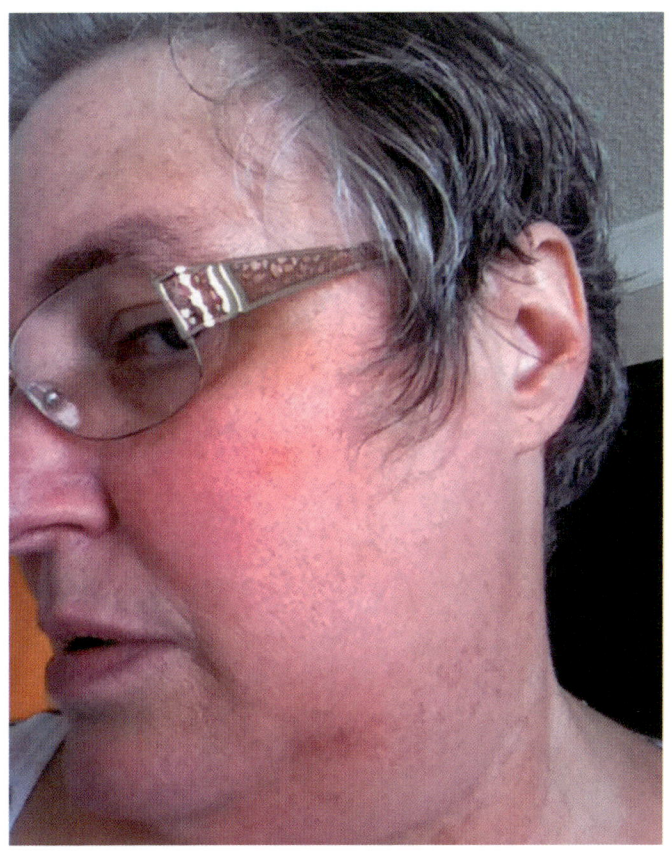

REDNESS

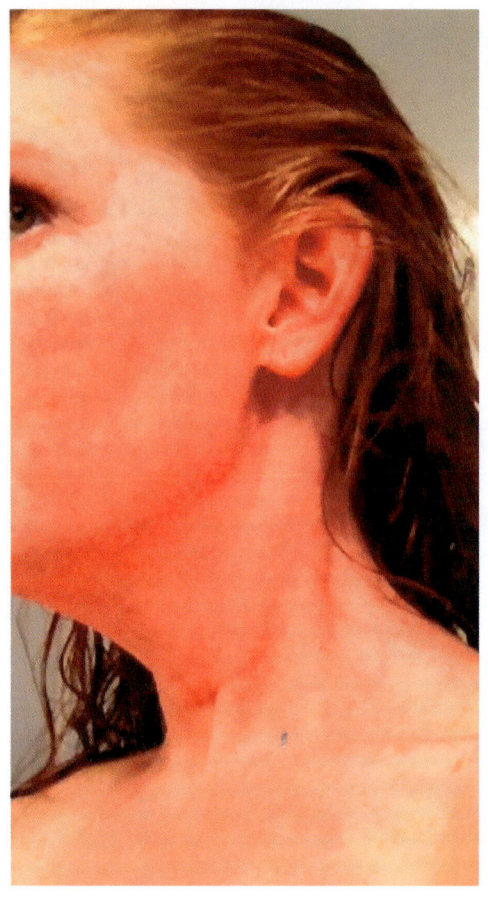

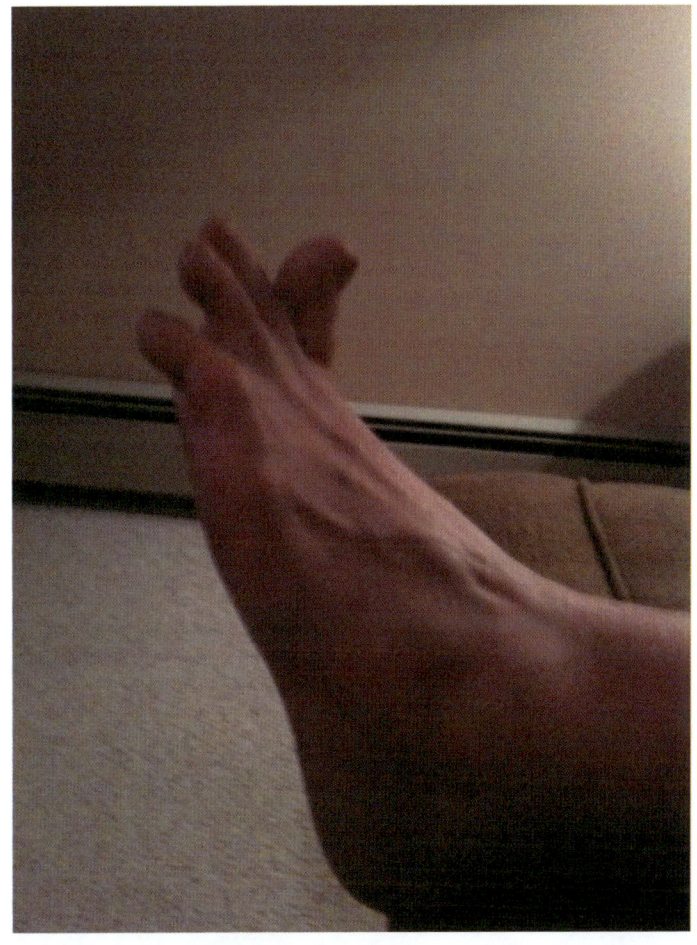

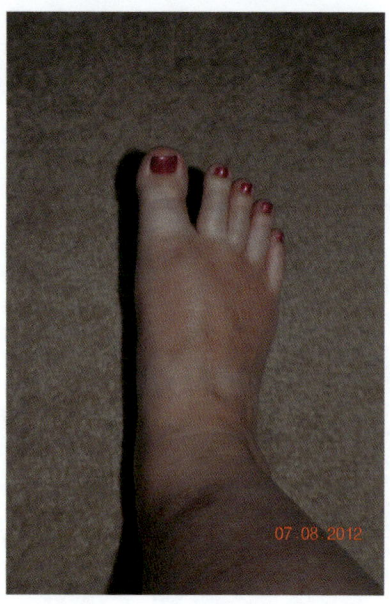

Distonia of the hand.

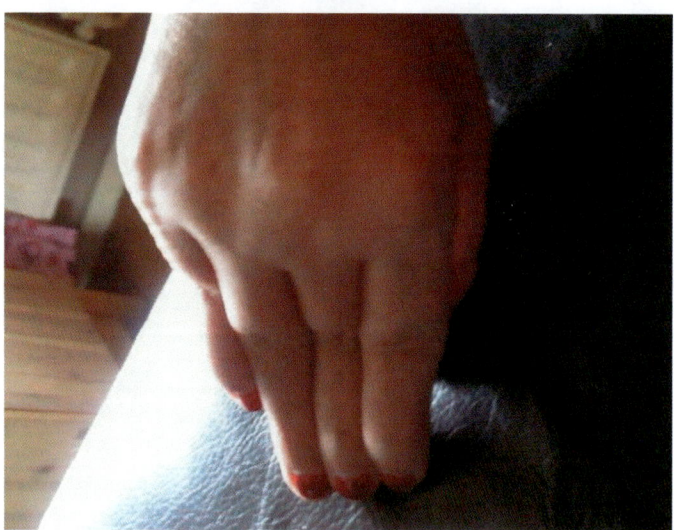

autonomic nervous system (ANS). The second is the so
Burning pain is the most common symptom. Some
descriptions of how it feels are that it is the worst sunburn

that you can imagine one thousand fold. Other describe it as if liter fluid were poured on them and lit by a match. Burning pain is associated with nerve pain. It is not exclusive to RSD but is a defining symptom of the disease.

Changes in the muscles and bone also occur. The muscles atrophy. The bones become more brittle. Many people experience dystonia. Dystonia is defined as a neurological movement disorder, in which sustained muscle contractions cause twisting, repetitive movements or abnormal postures. Pain causes lack of motion and lack of motion leads to atrophy. Dystonia further adds to immobility and if not treated can be devastating to the person with RSD causing them to be bedridden. Finally changes in the nails often take place. The nails thicken and become brittle. They often have ridges.

In order to understand the symptoms of CRPS, we need to take a step backwards and take a look at the central nervous system (CNS). Our CNS (central nervous system) is divided into to branches. The first is the autonomic nervous system (ANS). When we are talking about CRPS, our focus is on the ANS. The ANS is divided into two systems: the Parasympathetic Nervous System (PNS) and the Sympathetic Nervous System (SNS). The parasympathetic nervous system and the sympathetic nervous system work together to maintain homeostasis (a balance). When we look at the name Reflex Sympathetic Dystrophy, you see that it involves the sympathetic nervous system. RSD involves a sympathetic nervous system that is not operating correctly.

The autonomic nervous system (made up of the sympathetic and parasympathetic nervous systems) is responsible for the regulation of our internal organs. The ANS operates without any conscious effort on our part. ANS controls things like breathing, digestion, sweating, temperature control and our heart rate. We have little control over these functions. The sympathetic nervous system can cause things like our heart beating faster, our blood vessels dilating and our bronchi in the lungs dilating. The sympathetic nervous system is also known as the fight or flight system. When we are in danger, our sympathetic nervous system can cause our heart to beat faster, blood vessels and air pathways in the lungs to dilate. When working correctly, this gives a burst of energy that allows us to instinctively either fight or flee. Emotions such as fear, excitement and anger are caused by the sympathetic nervous system. Although the parasympathetic nervous system is not directly affected by CRPS, it works in opposition to the sympathetic nervous system to lower your heart rate, constrict your blood vessels and small airway tubules.

If your sympathetic nervous system is malfunctioning, you get an imbalance between the SNS and PNS. Without the trigger of danger your heart rate increases, blood vessels dilate, the tubules in your lungs dilate, you sweat, and can feel anxious, angry or fearful. By understanding what the sympathetic nervous system works, you can better understand the symptoms of CRPS.

In the beginning, the pain of CRPS is maintain by the sympathetic nervous system. Over time, the pain of CRPS becomes centralized. With the constant stimulation by pain signals in the CNS, the activation of the NMDA receptor occurs. Once the MNDA receptors are activated, the pain of CRPS is centralized.

CHAPTER 3
TREATMENT OPTIONS

No matter what type of treatment option(s) you and your physician decide on, it is important that it is an informed decision. This means that you have researched the treatment. You know the risks and benefits of the treatment for someone with CRPS You need to know how often your physician has performed this treatment and what their success rate is. Knowledge is power. There is very little about this disease that we have control over except for our ability to educate ourselves about CRPS, its treatment options and to chose our health care professionals carefully.

Medications
There is a Golden Rule for pain medications. The good must outweigh the bad. The effectiveness of the pain relief must outweigh the side effects from the medication. There should be an improvement in pain on a daily basis. If this doesn't happen, then the medication you are on is not right for you.   You should be on the lowest dosage of the medication that provides meaningful relief. There are several types of medications that are used to treat RSD pain.

Oral Medications –There are several classifications of medications that are used in the treatment of CRPS. They include but are not limited to anticonvulsants (medication that prevents seizures) anti-depressants (medication that treats depression) narcotics and opioids. Although it is impossible to list every medication used; here is an over view.

Anti-inflammatory medications often referred to as NSAIDs (Non-Steroidal Anti-inflammatory Drugs) and steroids help to reduce the inflammation associated with CRPS and offer some pain relief. Some researchers hypothesize that the anti-inflammatory components in NSAIDs are critical to the development or perpetuation of CRPS. Some theorize that CRPS is an inflammatory process within the nervous system.

Thus the use of anti-inflammatory drugs can slow the CRPS process. These medications can be used both during acute pain and as long-acting agents, known as prophylactics (preventatives). One theory is that if NSAIDs are used early and often, NSAIDs can be quite effective. In addition to treating CRPS, NSAIDs have also been used to treat other neuropathic pain conditions, particularly those associated with considerable inflammation. NSAIDs work by preventing the synthesis of prostaglandins, which mediate inflammation and hyperalgesia (hypersensitivity). In addition to their peripheral anti-inflammatory action, NSAIDs may also block spinal nociceptive processing (the processing of pain within the spinal cord). Some NSAID drugs may be more effective than others. Ketoprofen, for example offers substantial anti-inflammatory effects over some of the other NSAIDS. Oral steroids are strong anti-inflammatories but are normally not used long term but rather for flare ups. The potential side effects of both NSAIDs and steroids are not limited to stomach discomfort, bleeding, and in some cases have shown to precipitate heart attacks in those who are high risk. Risk factors include but are not limited to; heart disease, high cholesterol or in people who have had a stroke or previous heart attack.

 Anti-convulsant drugs (seizure medications) are used as prophylactic (preventative) agents in neuropathic pain. Anticonvulsants work by a variety of mechanisms thought to be relevant in the treatment of CRPS. Some block sodium and calcium channels, producing a decrease in neuron excitability. When the nerves are less excitable, they produce less electrical impulses reducing nerve pain as well as seizures. Gabapentin (aka Neurontin), is widely used for neuropathic pain. It first came to the attention of the research community when an anecdotal report touted its effect in the treatment of CRPS. The mechanism of action of Gabapentin is not completely understood. Other anti-convulsants being used in addition to Gabapentin are Topiramate (aka Topamax) which is not only used to treat CRPS but as a preventative medication for migraines that many with CRPS have. Side effects include but are not limited to sedation (often given at bedtime to enhance sleep), changes in the blood, and nystagmus (a searching movement of the eyes), tremor and incoordination.

Antidepressants are a traditional choice in neuropathic conditions. Heterocyclic antidepressants (HCAs) are used exclusively as maintenance agents. These antidepressants negatively react with many medications and some foods. Newer antidepressants such as the selective serotonin reuptake inhibitors (SSRIs) and serotonin-norpinephrin reutake inhibitors (SNRIs) have fewer side effects and are prescribed more frequently for depression but are not effective for chronic pain. Some better known HCAs are Amitriptyline (Elivil), Desipramine (Norpramin) Doxepin (Silenor,Zonalon), Imipramine (Tofranil) and Noriptyline (Aventyl, Pamelor). They are often used in lower dosages to treat chronic pain than when used to treat depression. Side effects are individual to each of the antidepressants but common side effects are dry mouth, dizziness, drowsiness (thus often prescribed at bedtime to help with sleep), headache, weight gain and constipation. You should never stop taking these medications suddenly or without the knowledge of your physician. Stopping them suddenly can have serious consequences.

Opioids An opioid is a chemical that works by binding to opioid receptors, which are found principally in the central and peripheral nervous system as well as the gastrointestinal tract. The receptors in these organ systems mediate both the beneficial effects and the side effects of opioids.The analgesic effects of opioids are due to decreased perception of pain, decreased reaction to pain as well as increased pain tolerance. Opioids are well known for their ability to produce a feeling of euphoria, motivating some to recreationally use opioids.

Although the term opiate is often used as a synonym for narcotics, the term opiate is properly limited to the natural alkaloids found in the resin of the opium poppy (The poppy is a flower). In some definitions, the semi-synthetic substances that are directly derived from the opium poppy are considered to be opiates as well, while in other classification systems these substances are simply referred to as semi-synthetic opioids. Use of opioids for chronic pain management is still subject to some controversy. For the most part, neuropathic pain does not respond to opioids as well as nociceptive pain does. It is for this reason that neuropathic pain requires higher doses. With higher doses also comes an increase in the risks of side effects. When used for chronic pain long acting agents should be used for maintenance of chronic pain and as a short-acting agent for acute need. It often takes larger dosages of opioids for the recipient to receive the same result. It has been shown that opioids lower the pain threshold. The side effects of opioids include but are not limited to; a feeling of euphoria, nausea and vomiting, drowsiness, itching, dry mouth, headache, and constipation.

Opioids trigger the activation of glia cells. For someone with CRPS they are counter productive because the activation of glia cells causes an increase in inflammation and pain.

For more information on glia cells and the role that they play in CRPS go to YouTube and search Nancy Cotterman. There you will find presentations by leading CRPS physicians.

Methadone may have a special place in the treatment of CRPS because of its NMDA antagonist. As mentioned in the previous chapter, the activation of the NMDA receptors is what causes the CRPS pain to become centralized. These drugs attach to the MNDA receptors and block them. NMDA receptor antagonists are a class of anesthetics that work to inhibit the action of, the N-methyl d-aspartate receptor (NMDAR). They are used more commonly in veterinary medicine. They are known as dissociative anethesetic (causing an out of body feeling). Several synthetic opioids function additionally as NMDAR-antagonists, such as Meperidine, Methadone, Dextropropoxyphene, Tramadol and Ketobemidone, Ketamine (K), Dextromethorphan (DXM), Phencyclidine (PCP), and Nitrous Oxide (N2O aka laughing gas). These drugs are popular as recreational drugs for their dissociative, hallucinogenic, and/or euphoriant properties,.

Narcotics Not all narcotics are opioids but many do fall into that classification. A narcotic is a classification of medication used for pain management. Some individuals define narcotics as those substances that bind at opiate receptors (cellular membrane proteins activated by substances like heroin or morphine) while others refer to any illicit substance as a narcotic. In a legal context, narcotic refers to opium, opium derivatives, and their semi-synthetic substitutes. For the purposes of this discussion, the term narcotic refers to drugs that produce morphine-like effects.

Narcotics are used therapeutically to treat pain, suppress cough, alleviate diarrhea, and induce anesthesia. Narcotics are administered in a variety of ways. Some are taken orally, transdermally (skin patches), or injected (either into a muscle or into a vein). They are also available in suppositories. Drug effects depend heavily on the dose, route of administration, and previous exposure to the drug. Aside from their medical use, narcotics produce a general sense of well-being by reducing tension, anxiety, and aggression. These effects are helpful in a therapeutic setting but can contribute to their abuse.

Narcotic use is associated with a variety of unwanted effects including drowsiness, inability to concentrate, apathy, lessened physical activity, constriction of the pupils, dilation of the subcutaneous blood vessels causing flushing of the face and neck, constipation, nausea and vomiting, and most significantly, respiratory depression. As the dose is increased, the subjective analgesic (pain relief), and toxic effect become more pronounced. Except in cases of acute intoxication, there is no loss of motor coordination or slurred speech as occurs with many depressants.

Anti-hypertensives and a-adrenergic antagonists
Clonidine is an α-adrenergic agonist (it works similarly to

epinephrin which regulates the heart rate, diameter of the blood vessels and air passages, it initiates our fight or flight response) that is often used for the treatment of RSD by enhancing the effects of pain medications. By enhancing the effect of pain medication, the patient can be on a lower dose It is used orally, in patch form (transdermal) and epiduraly (drugs are delivered into the epidural space in the spine) to treat "sympathetically maintained pain". Sympathetically maintained pain is pain that caused by the sympathetic nervous system) Case studies have shown that transdermal Clonidine could reduce or eliminate local CRPS-induced hyperalgesia (increase in response to painful stimulus) and allodynia (painful response to normal stimulus) Nifedipine, a calcium channel blocker, has been shown to be effective in the management of symptoms sometimes associated with RSD (ex, for control of intense vasoconstriction).

Phenoxybenzamine and Phentolamine are nonselective α-adrenergic antagonists (suppresses the fight or flight response) that some have suggested for CRPS. There is also support for the use of oral Phenoxybenzamine, which seems to have an optimal effect in CRPS that is less than 3 months in duration.

Low Dose Naltrexone (LND) Originally Naltrexone was developed and approved by the FDA for helping heroin or opium addicts by blocking the effects of these drugs. In low dosages (4.5 – 6 mg per day) it has been shown to activate ones own endorphins (our internal opioids) and lower pain. Our endorphins also play a positive central role in the orchestration of our immune system. Many people with CRPS have a compromised immune system. One side effect of LND can be insomnia. It is usually taken in the morning. The insomnia usually subsides over time. For additional information on LDN go to YouTube and search Pradeep Chopra, MD.

Topical Preparations Topical treatments for CRPS differ from transdermal medications (patches) like the Fentanyl or Clonidine patch because they only allow for absorption of the medication locally to the affected skin and soft tissue area. Topical treatments for RSD include the 5% lidocaine patch, the Eutectic Mixture of Local Anesthetics (EMLA) cream, Capsaicin and DiMethylSulfOxide (DMSO). There is some literature endorsing the use of EMLA for patients with RSD. It is used to numb the area prior to an IV stick, blood draw or injection. The lidocaine patch is a non-woven patch containing 5% lidocaine; it is FDA-approved for the management of postherpetic (herpies) neuralgia, and is used increasingly for RSD. This formulation of lidocaine does not produce any anesthesia but rather only analgesia (pain relief). It is effective in treating allodynia. (painful response to normal stimuli). Capsaicin, a compound found in chili peppers, frequently provokes a painful burning sensation at the site of application and therefore is not an effective treatment for a person with RSD. DMSO helps medication absorb into the skin. It has anti-inflammatory effects as well as blocking nerve stimulus. In one study DMSO (50% cream used for two months) showed significant pain reduction when compared with a placebo. It is often used as the base in compounded creams that physicians prescribe to be used topically. These creams can be compounded using other medications that are effective in treating the neuropathic pain such as Clonidine, Neurontin, Lidocaine and Ketamine. Many doctors treating RSD have a favorite combination of drugs that they have compounded with DSMO as the base of the cream.

A word of caution; if you are using compounded creams or other topical compounds, you need to be sure that you wash your hands thoroughly before touching young children or pets. The cream may transfer to the child or pet. Be sure that your pet doesn't lick the area where you have applied the cream. If you have any concerns, please contact your physician and/or veterinarian.

Transdermal Medications Some medications are formulated into transdermal patches. These patches allow for continuous and uniform absorption of the medication through the blood vessels in the skin. Some examples of transdermal medications are Fentynl Patches (an opioid drug), and Clonidine Patch. They offer a more uniform relief than their oral counterparts.

Intravenous Medications Many of the previously mentioned oral medications are also available in intravenous (IV) form. These include the opioids, Lidocaine, hypertensive and a-adrenergic antagonists (suppress the fight or flight response). Another classification of IV medications are the MNDA inhibitors. The most widely used over the past decade is Ketamine (on the street known as special K).

Ketamine is a dissociative anesthesia (it can cause an out of body feeling). It has been used in veterinary medicine and prior to the invention of anesthesia with less side effects It was also used as a general anesthesia for surgery. Over the past decade, there have been countless studies on Ketamine and neuropathic pain including RSD. (There will be links listed to some of these studies in Appendix G) Ketamine acts to reboot the nervous system. Ketamine is a noncompetitive NMDA receptor (NMDAR) antagonist which means that Ketamine's actions interfere with pain transmission in the spinal cord. Ketamine also inhibits nitric oxide synthase, inhibiting production of nitric oxide, a neurotransmitter involved in pain perception, and therefor further contributing to analgesia. Ketamine binds to the opioid receptors. Many physicians feel that the Ketamine recipient must be off of all opioids due to the fact that the opioids block the Ketamine from acting on the opioid receptors and thus reducing the effectiveness of the Ketamine.

Ketamine is given in four ways:
Coma Ketamine At the writing of this book (12/31/13), coma Ketamine is not available. Between 2001 and 2011 in Germany and Mexico patients were put into a Ketamine drug induced coma for six days. A breathing tube and invasive monitoring were required to keep the patient stable during this treatment.

Hospital-based infusions The hospital-based infusions require a five to six day in-patient stay, usually in an ICU

32

(Intensive Care Unit) . An intravenous (IV) line is inserted and the patient is started on a dose of 10 mg of ketamine per hour,. The dosage is increased by 10 mg increments until the patient feels "tipsy". The dose is then maintained at that dose for the duration of the treatment (five or six days). In addition, Clonidine, 0.1 mg (per FDA) is administered along with small doses of Lorazepam (Ativan®), 1-to-2 mg, and Versed (2 - 4 mgs) for any feelings of anxiety or hallucinations. Other medications are utilized to treat such problems, included but not limited to nausea, vomiting and headache. During the infusion blood work is done daily. The hospital monitors your heart rhythm, blood pressure and oxygen saturation.

Following discharge from the hospital, patients typically enroll in an outpatient infusion program of varying degrees and lengths. Dr Robert J Schwartzman of Drexel University in Philadelphia is responsible for developing the outpatient infusion protocol (often referred to as boosters) The protocol starts with two consecutive outpatient infusions two weeks after discharge from the hospital. Two weeks later, a four hour infusion is given on two consecutive days. One month later, a four hour infusion is given on two consecutive days. After this, boosters are give as four hour infusions on two consecutive days every two to three months as a maintenance plan.During the out patient infusions nurses monitor your heart rhythm, blood pressure and oxygen saturation. There are variations of this protocol.

Outpatient 10 day protocol Many insurance companies will not cover the inpatient Ketamine and there are fewer doctors able to do the inpatient protocol. The outpatient 10 protocol is a viable alternative. This protocol was also established by Dr Robert J Schwartzman of Drexel University (who retired in June of 2013) These patients are given therapy only on an outpatient basis. The infusions are administered in a outpatient infusion suite. The physician administers a four hour infusion of ketamine per day Monday through Friday on two consecutive weeks. During the out patient infusions nurses monitor your heart rhythm, blood pressure and oxygen saturation.

After completion of the 10 day outpatient protocol, patients are placed in the maintenance outpatient program (boosters) as described above. There have been few adverse reactions to Ketamine infusions. The most common side effects are, nausea during/after the infusion, fatigue and a headache. There have been no documented long term side effects. Most patients are given 2 mg of Midazolam (Versed) and sleep through the infusion. Other medications are given as needed for side effects such as nausea and headache. There have been instances of bladder issues in those that abuse Ketamine on a daily basis but to date this has not developed in patients managed as above.

I'd like to give you a brief history of Ketamine in the US. In 2001, it was hoped that a Ketamine induced coma would cure CRPS. Ketamine blocks the MNDA receptors. It did prove to bring many a reduction in their symptoms. Over time the symptoms returned in most people. I was part of a study conducted in Germany in coordination with a CRPS specialist in the US. I was the fifth person to travel to Germany in this study to be put into a Ketamine induced coma. Over time, the coma protocol was refined to prevent hallucinations and dissociative side effects. Drugs such as Versed, Fentynl and Clonopin were added to the IV mix. The dosage of Ketamine was based on the patients weight. This required ICU care. In 2001, there was no follow up once the study participants returned to the US. For most, the symptoms slowly returned. In February of 2002, an outpatient low dose infusion program was set up and there were two of us who began this program. After a while there was in increase in the number of people participating in the coma study. This follow up treatment became another study. In this treatment we were given a Ketamine infusion over four hours. Drs Schwartzman and Goldberg worked to find what dose and what length of time (number of days consecutively) were needed to reduce our symptoms once again. We were awake during this treatment. This treatment became known as Ketamine boosters. Patients who had not participated in the coma study were added to the outpatient Ketamine program in the US. That became the 10 day protocol. At the same time, another doctor was studying a protocol that he learned when studying in Australia. This protocol involved a 24/7 low dose awake infusion that was done in the hospital. In this protocol the Ketamine was titrated up slowly until the person began to feel drunk. The dosage was leveled off at this rate. In addition to the Ketamine, Versed and Clonopin were given to help with the side effects of the Ketamine. In recent years, some anesthesiologists felt that it was the strength of the dosage that was important and not the length of time in which it was infused. At this time, this controversy still exists. With all of the present day infusions the potential side effects include hallucinations, dizziness, headache, and fatigue. Versed given in adequate dosages prevents the hallucinations. Zophran is given before and after the infusion to reduce nausea and Toradol is given to prevent the headache. Some of the side effects such as headache are actually related to the Versed and not the Ketamine.

When deciding if Ketamine infusions are the right treatment for you, you should research the treatment itself. You should inquire about the results of the physician administering the infusion has attained. You need to decide whether or not outpatient infusions (either high dose or low dose) or inpatient infusions are right for you. Prior to either of these options, blood work, a psychological evaluation and often an EKG need to be done prior to the treatment. The exact preKetamine tests ordered vary from physician to physician. With all of these different Ketamine infusions you will have blood pressure monitoring, EKG (heart) monitoring and oxygen monitoring. If you have a reduction in pain from the Ketamine infusion the length of time that it lasts will vary from person to person. Additional Ketamine infusions (boosters) are often required. (see appendix G for more information on Ketamine infusions).

An older but effective infusion therapy for CRPS is Lidocaine. Lidocaine Infusions: Lidocaine is a medication that many of you may associate as a numbing agent like novocaine or as a drug used in the treatment of heart arrhythmias . For CRPS, intravenous Lidocaine is administered in an escalating dose over five days. The Lidocaine dosage is increased until the blood level is at the range that the doctor wants (a therapeutic level). The dosage is then leveled off to maintain that blood level over the five days. This requires daily blood tests to monitor the blood level of the Lidocaine. During the infusion your blood pressure, EKG (heart) and oxygen saturation are closely monitored. The Lidocaine is mixed with an IV solution and infused on a pump. Possible side effects include a drop in blood pressure, cardiac arrhythmia, dysphoria and dizziness. The purpose of the infusion is to decrease pain and allodynia. Often the RSD symptoms return; the length of time varies from person to person. If the treatment is successful in improving the persons symptoms, the infusion can be repeated as out patient boosters just as with the Ketamine. Articles on Lidocaine infusions can be found in Appendix G.

With both Lidocaine and Ketamine infusions IV access can be an issue. Many with CRPS have poor veins or have had so many IV sticks that their veins are scared. You add the fact that IV sticks can not only cause flare ups and even a spread in the CRPS. Many physicians believe that a more permanent IV access is needed for the frequent infusions. See Appendix N for information on the different types of IV access.

Medication Storage – Whether or not you have children at home, you need to be responsible for keeping your medications in a safe place. You never store medications in the bathroom medicine cabinet for two reasons. First the dampness and increased temperature that occur in the bathroom are harmful for the medications. Secondly anyone who uses your bathroom has access to them. You should purchase a small safe. They make them in all sizes. You should keep the safe or lock box locked and keep the key in a safe place. Even if you are not on opioids, if taken improperly, ány medication can be harmful to a child, pet or adult. Keep the safe in a dry place.

When you travel, you should carry your mediations with you.

Do not check them in your luggage or leave them in the car. Your medications should be kept in their original containers from the drug store. Carrying medications in a medication dispenser is not a good idea. If traveling by air, you may not be permitted to go through security if your medication is not in its original container.

Medication Disposal – Please don't flush unused medications down the toilet. This gets into the water table and can affect our drinking water. Many pharmacies have a take back program for expired or extra medications. If you do not have a program like this in your area then take some coffee grounds and put the unused medication into the coffee grounds. Place the medication and coffee grounds into a plastic bag. You can then throw them in the trash. Don't just throw your empty medication bottles in the trash. If someone goes through your trash, they will have your name and address and they will know what medications you are on. Remove the label from the bottle before you dispose of it.

Therapies: PT, OT, Aqua Therapy –
Physical Therapy – Physical therapy can be beneficial in helping to keep the person with RSD moving; however it should not be done to excess. In other words, strenuous physical therapy can cause more harm than good. When choosing a physical therapist, be sure that they understand RSD and have worked with others with CRPS. If they have no CRPS experience then they can do more harm.

Occupational Therapy – Occupational Therapy's goal is to help you with the activities of daily living (ADL). This can be very beneficial of you are having difficulty using one of your limbs. They can help the person with RSD find different ways to do everyday things. Once again, you do not want to see an OT who has not worked with people with CRPS before and don't have a good understanding of the disease.

With both PT and OT, you will be taught exercises to continue at home. It is important for the person with RSD to keep moving as much as possible to prevent atrophy.hey offer ultrasound therapy, massage, tens units and other modalities that can be helpful in getting the RSD patient to move. It is important that you keep moving to help prevent muscle atrophy and joint freezing.

Therapeutic Aqua Therapy – Warm water (90 – 94 degrees) can be the perfect atmosphere to start moving. For most, the warm water itself is soothing. Exercising in water makes you more buoyant and takes the weight off of sore joints. Once again, Aqua Therapy can be over done. It should be taken slowly and the therapist should have a knowledge of CRPS. Aqua therapy works great in conjunction with Ketamine, Lidocaine or Opioid treatments. These medications decrease the pain and allows the person with CRPS to move again. A great place to start rehabbing and get movement back again is in a therapeutic pool.

Multidisciplinary Chronic Pain Programs – There are rehabilitation hospitals and pain centers that offer a multidisciplinary approach to CRPS minimizing or eliminating the use of medications. These programs often offer individual psychological therapy, group therapy, biofeedback, the use of relaxation to deal with pain, physical therapy and occupational therapy.

Biofeedback is the process of becoming aware of your pain and bodily functions using instrumentations that provide information on your bodies functions. With the process you learn to control things like your brainwaves, muscle tone, skin conductance, heart rate and pain. Eventually you learn how to control these functions without the use of the machine. It is an effective tool in managing your pain and can be used in combination with other treatments.

Hyperbaric Oxygen Therapy (HBOT) – This is a treatment that is used when a diver comes up to quickly and gets the bends. It is also used in wound healing. The patient is put into a chamber and high concentrations of oxygen are administered. The patient usually has multiple days of this therapy. There are mixed reviews as to whether this is helpful to the CRPS patient. Most physicians do not see it as a viable treatment as there is no evidence that increasing your oxygen levels can decrease the pain of CRPS or reverse the damage that it may have caused. Insurance does not cover HBOT for CRPS.

Calmare is a non-invasive, non-pharmaceutical solution for pain control and drug resistant pain. It uses biophysical "scrambler" technology, a type of treatment for nerve pain that uses electrodes placed on the skin. Very low doses of electricity are transmitted from the electrodes through the to block the pain. A series of calmare sessions are done on consecutive days. If you have a spinal column stimulator this treatment is contraindicated. Insurance does not pay for this. The treatment involves stimulation of nerves that are already hyper-stimulated. Most reputable CRPS physicians do not recommend this treatment.

Blocks
Many blocks are done with continuous x-ray (fluoroscopy) and under some sort of sedation. There are two main types of blocks.

Sympathetic Blocks - There a whole host of sympathetic blocks depending on the area being treated. The one thing that they have in common is that medication is injected, using a needle, into a specific area with the intent of blocking sympathetic mediated pain (pain caused by the sympathetic nervous system) The length of time that relief is felt varies from person to person and based on the skill of your practitioner. Some practitioners only inject an anethesetic only such as Marcaine. Others mix the anesthetic with a steroid such as Depot. Too many Depot injections can cause Cushing Syndrome which is the production of too much cortisol. It can cause elevated blood sugar levels and other complications. Some examples of sympathetic blocks include: Bier Block (of the foot), Lumbar Sympathetic Block (done in the lumbar region of the back) and Occipital Blocks (done in the occipital region of the head). Depending on the source of your pain, a sympathetic block can be done in an associated region of the body. Some practitioners use the sympathetic block as a diagnostic tool. They feel that if you respond to the block then in fact you have CRPS and if you do not respond then you do not have CRPS. The problem is that not everyone with CRPS responds to sympathetic blocks. Some people even get a flare in their pain from them so this is not considered a good diagnostic tool. Sympathetic blocks can be done in combination with other treatments such as oral medications, IV infusions, and trigger point injections. It is part of a multi-treatment plan. The concern with sympathetic blocks is that the needle is placed near nerves and blood vessels. It is a possibility that the needle could cause damage to the nerve or blood vessel. Once the pain is centralized, sympathetic blocks are of no use.

Trigger Point Injections – A trigger point injection (TPI) is an injection into painful points of the body. Trigger points are discrete, focal hyper irritable spots (places that cause pain upon touch) located in a tense band of skeletal muscle. For the person with CRPS these hyper-irritable points add to the persons pain. With the TPI these places are palpated and marked with a surgical marker. The practitioner may use a dry needle (not inject any medication) or may inject an anesthetic such as Marcaine or an anesthetic steroid mixture such as Marcaine and Depot. At first, these areas may be more painful than before the injection but as the anesthetic begins to work the area becomes numb. This numbness is short lived and some people once again experience an increase in pain from irritation from the steroid. Once the steroid begins to do its job, the result should be a relief from the pain as the muscle is no longer inflamed and tense. Trigger point injections can be in combination with sympathetic blocks, oral medication, IV infusions and other treatments. It is rarely done as a single treatment for CRPS but rather part of a multi-treatment approach to care. The risk here is that needle sticks have been linked to the cause of CRPS and to the spread of CRPS. You and your physician need to weigh the potential benefits agains the potential risks.

Epidural – An epidural can be a series of single injections or a continuous infusion of a numbing medication. The placement of the epidural depends on where your CRPS is. Most people have heard of epidurals and associate them with childbirth. The single injection protocol are injections of an anethesetic (sometimes mixed with a steroid) into the epidural space in the spinal column at a specific level on the spine. This is normally done under continuous x-ray (fluoroscopy) so that the physician can see exactly where he/she wants to place the needle. Most of the time you are sedated for the procedure so that you feel nor remember anything. An IV is started to administer these sedating medications. You can not eat or drink after midnight prior to the procedure. Side effects can include bleeding and infection from the introduction of a needle. Once the sedation wears off, you can go home within an hour of the procedure with someone else driving. Sedation is not always done; it is up to the discretion of the practitioner and a question that you would want to ask your practitioner prior to agreeing to an epidural with them.

A continuous epidural is normally done in the hospital. A numbing medication is infused via a pump like the pump that they use for IVs and disperses a continuous flow of medication. When the epidural is done in the lower back, your legs are numb and you feel no pain for the time that the epidural is being infused. It is used to give you a break from the pain and to calm down the pain so that when the infusion is over, hopefully your pain level is lower. Epidurals that are done continuously in the hospital can run for up to a week. You will have an IV and your vital signs will be monitored. Side effects include a drop in blood pressure, infection and bleeding from the insertion of the catheter that it is left in place during the infusion, headache and spinal fluid leakage. This procedure will not eliminate CRPS but rather is a comfort measure.

Surgical Options

Medication pump – A.K.A. Intrathecal Pump One form of treatment is the medication pump. With this implanted devise a small pump, about the size of a hockey puck is placed in the lower abdomen. A catheter is tunneled under the skin and placed the intrathecal space in the spinal canal. This space is further into the spinal canal than the epidural space. A battery is contained within the pump as well as a reservoir that can contain medications. The pump pushes the medication through the catheter into the intrathecal space in your spine where it is dispersed and bathes the nerves within the spinal cord. (photos in appendix D)

Before you would be considered for this surgery, a trial would be done to see if this treatment works for you. A catheter is placed into your spine and hooked to and external pump. The medication that you physician is considering using is placed into an external pump and infused into the intrathecal space in your back. Your physician may try a combination of medications or different separate medications. If you respond well to the trial, then you will have the option of moving forward with the surgery. This surgery is usually done by a neurosurgeon or pain management physician. Be sure that you meet with the physician before the surgery and get all of your questions answers answered.
For a synopsis of what the surgery is like see appendix D.

When you have the surgery, it is usually done as a same day surgery. You will have an incision on your abdomen. A small pocket is made in your abdomen to the side of your umbilicus. The pocket is made above the muscle just under the skin to hold the pump itself. There is a catheter that runs from the pump to your back through a tunnel that is made under your skin. There will be bruising where they tunnel the catheter to the back where you will have a second incision. They anchor the catheter and place it into the intrathecal space in your spinal column through the incision in your back. Here are two photos of what my incisions looked like after my medication pump surgery. You will be quite sore as you will have incisions on your abdomen and your back along with bruising on your one side.

So, what are the risks of the medication pump? First of all there are the risks of the surgery which are infection, spinal fluid leak, bleeding and headache. There are also the anesthesia risks. There is a risk of CRPS spread from the surgery. There is also the slight risk of infection every time that the pump is refilled. The pump could move under the skin and cause damage. The catheter can dislodge at any point and cause a spinal fluid leak. The pump could stop functioning causing the medication to stop infusing into the intrathecal space causing a sudden withdrawal from the medication   Some people experience extreme pain with the pump in the pocket that is made right under the skin in the abdomen due to a RSD reaction. Some people can not tolerate the feel of the pump in their body and have to have it removed. For me, that was not the case. In my case, the battery failed, which in 2001 was an issue for this company but has not been a problem since too my knowledge. This did cause a sudden withdrawal of the morphine and I became very sick. I did not know that the battery had failed. I went to a local hospital that did not deal with the pump. I had just had the pump filled two days before so none of us even gave it a thought that this was the cause of my violent vomiting and diarrhea. I was hospitalized for 6 days for dehydration and to stop the vomiting and diarrhea. It wasn't until I returned to the physician who managed my pump that we found out that it had stopped working. The symptoms that I experienced was morphine withdrawal.

Narcotics, such as Morphine can be placed into the pump as can anti-spasmodic medications such as Baclofin or a combination of medications. The pump is programed via computer with a radio frequency wand placed externally over the pump by a specially trained nurse and doctor. The pump is refilled by a specially trained nurse or doctor.

A smaller amount of medication is needed to get the same response compared to oral medication; however it takes can still require increasing amount of intrathecal medication to get the same response to pain. The benefit is that you don't get the peaks and valleys in medication levels that you get when taking the medication by mouth. With the pump, you are receiving a continuous flow of medication. Additionally, the pump can be programmed to give an increased dosage during times of the day that are known to be bad pain times of day for the person with RSD and less medication during times of the day that are known to be good times of the day.

My personal experience with the pump – When the pump was operating, I did experience the need for increasing dosages to get the same effect. I was drossy all of the time from the Morphine in addition to Clonidine. I didn't feel that the Morphine really helped with the burning nerve pain but did help with the aching bone pain that lingered from the multiple fractures to my foot. At the time that I had this device implanted; there weren't many options available and I was still of the mind set that I needed to find a solution to put and end to this pain. I hadn't yet accepted that this was something that I would have to live with and adapt my life to.

If you are considering a medication pump, you need to look at the pros and cons of this treatment. If a specific medication is working for you and it is able to be delivered intrathecally then this may be a good solution. If you feel that you are a good candidate for and can receive Ketamine with the surgery for the person and you are willing to commit to the regular care of the device; then perhaps this device is the right thing for you, Just like everyones CRPS is different, everyones treatment needs to be tailored to fit their CRPS.

Spinal Column Stimulator (SCS) – a spinal column stimulator is a device that has electrical leads that are placed in the spine (cervical, thoracic or lumbar) to stimulate different areas of the spinal column. The device gives you a tingling feeling in the targeted area. The theory behind it is like when you have a bug bite that itches and you slap it, the pain from the slap stops the perception of the itching. The tingling sent through the nerve blocks the perception of the pain in the targeted area.(See appendix P for photos). Again like calamare, the SCS stimulates already hyper–stimulated nerves. Even if you respond well to the trial, the effects of SCS are usually not long lasting.

This does involve surgery. The spinal column stimulator (SCS) is a surgically place device that is about the size of a stop watch. It sends mild electrical impulses to the epidural space near the spine through one or more thin wires, called leads. This electrical impulse causes the tingling feeling in the targeted area. The physician can program these leads so that they pulse in a specific way. The patient has a programer that is placed over the stimulator and allows the patient to increase or decrease the magnitude of the tingling and to turn the devise off and on. The handheld patient programmer allows you to make changes in the physician preprogramed settings within the stimulator.

Just like with the Intrathecal pump, a trial of the SCS is done to see if it is the right treatment for you. The leads that contain electrodes are placed on your spine. The wires are external and taped into place. They are attached to the external stimulator. You will be given the actual stimulator to be worn like a fanny pack. The patient is given a mini-programer so that the can adjust the stimulator to get the best relief. It works much like a TV remote control.

For people with CRPS, the stimulator is most effective if used early on as it does not is effective on sympathetically maintained pain (SMS). It doesn't work as well on Sympathetically Independent Pain (SIP or centralized pain), which is pain that is no longer maintained by the sympathetic nervous system . After the first year of CRPS, the pain changes from SMS to SIP. If the stimulator is placed in that first year, it will help with the CRPS pain for that first year. The decision here is is it worth the risks of surgery and a lengthy recovery for a potentially short term pain relief.

The risks of this procedure are the risks of the surgery include but are not limited to infection, bleeding, possible injury to the spine causing paralysis and anesthesia risks. The possible complications from the device itself are also infection, migration of the lead, and in some people sensitivity to the device itself.

Radio Ablations/Sympathectomies/Rysotomies – These procedures involve the removal or revision of the nerve(s) thought to be causing the CRPS. These are old procedures and should not be done. The nerve grows back and often the pain is worse once the nerve regrows.

Amputation There are still physicians that offer amputation of the affective limb as a treatment for CRPS. This absolutely should not be done. When a limb is amputated the person often experiences fantom limb pain. This burning pain is very similar to the pain of CRPS. Having CRPS makes someone more susceptible to phantom limb pain so now the person has the handicap of living with a missing limb and still has pain.

CHAPTER 4
FINANCES

Many people with CRPS can no longer work and those who do often have to modify their job to enable them to keep working.

Social Security Disability (SSD) The Social Security Administration passed a specific ruling regarding Reflex Sympathetic Dystrophy aka CRPS. Either terminology can be used in filing for SSD. You can find the ruling in Appendix A.

When you read it some of the treatments suggested in this ruling you will read about treatments that are no longer considered the Gold Standard of Medical Care; such as sympathectomies (which was mentioned in the treatment section). Ok, so what does all of that mean? Within the ruling, it outlines the documentation that will help them make their ruling. This is what you need to concentrate on in this ruling. Applying for SSD benefits can be a long and complicated process. Many get turned down on your first application.

Documentation needed: You should gather up all of the documentation (doctor's notes, procedures, tests, etc.) that you have on your illness. Arrange everything in a chronological order; doctor visits, sick leave episodes, diagnosis, treatments, medications, etc. Make at least 4 copies of each for your personal use, your attorney (if you chose to hire one), Social Security and your employer. Keeping a pain diary is also useful. For each day, write how you are feeling, your pain level, the medications that you took, and your pain level after the medication takes effect.

Check out the web site: http://www.ssa.gov/pgm/disability.htm

These are Social Security's criteria for applying on line for applying for disability benefits:

Review the Adult Disability Checklist
Complete the Disability Benefit Application
Complete the Adult Disability Report
Complete the Authorization to Disclose Information form (SSA-827). You can do this electronically as part of your Adult Disability Report or print and mail the form to your Social Security Office.
 Electronic Signature Process For Form SSA-827

Why Should I Apply Online?
Applying online for disability benefits offers several advantages:

*You can start your disability claim immediately. There is no need to wait for an appointment

*You can apply from the convenience of your own home or on any computer

*You avoid trips to a Social Security office, saving you time and money

Who Can Use The Online Application?

You can use the online application to apply for benefits if you:
*are age 18 or older;

*are not currently receiving benefits on your own Social Security record

*have worked and paid Social Security taxes long enough to qualify

*have a medical condition that has prevented you from working or is expected to prevent you from working for at least 12 months or end in death.

If you don't have computer access or are not comfortable applying on line, you can find the number for your local Social Security Offices in the Blue Pages of your phone book.

Since you have to be out of work for 12 months before being awarded SSD, you can not work at all during the 12 month period or the 12 months starts over again. If you employer offers short term and/or long term disability, it is advisable to apply for that as these benefits start right after you stop working. Although they most likely will not replace your full salary, they provide a set percentage. Check on any policies that your employer has on disability insurance. Check with the benefit's office of your employer to see if they offer COBRA for your health insurance if you are the one who holds your health insurance coverage.

It is advisable that you start compiling your documentation as soon as possible. Note that many doctors/hospital charge a copying fee. You can send them a request for your records in writing or via fax there is an example of a request for records form is in the Appendix B.

Social Security has very stringent guidelines, especially during the first two steps. Most people, no matter what the illness, lose in the first two steps. It is the third step that most cases are won. As a nurse, I am a documentation freak. Since I was involved in a personal injury law suit, I had to keep meticulous records for my attorney, including a journal. I actually won my case immediately. Documentation is everything. Don't be surprised if this process takes a year or longer.

If you have a close friend or family member who can work with you on this process it is very helpful. This process is very stressful and you really need the support of someone you are close to. If you case comes to a hearing, it is helpful if your support person understands your illness as they can be a great asset in a hearing.

Many of us put on a good front for friends and family members rather than expressing the amount of pain that we are actually in. DO NOT put on your normal act when in front of the judge. Let your real pain show through. Your mobility, or lack there of, how long you can stand, sit, do repetitive activities, how far you can walk, what you can lift and carry, your ability to concentrate, your dexterity, insomnia, sensitivity to tough, noise, light and sound, as well as your medications are the things that Social Security is looking at. When you describe your illness, think of yourself on your worst day.

Don't take for granted that your attorney or the judge is familiar with CRPS. Do some research and print out articles located in the appendix about CRPS so that you can provide them with proper information on CRPS. When you file your papers, enclosing a brochure from RSDSA.org or RSDHope.org that explains RSD is a good idea. If you are asked to provide ICD 10 codes for RSD, you will find them in the Appendix C

Workman's Compensation
If you were injured at work; it is your employer with the assistance of their workman's compensation insurance that will be covering your medical bills and salary. For this reason, if you are injured at work, it is important to report the injury immediately. If your employer has an injury form, fill it out as soon as you can. Often you need to hire a lawyer to represent you in order for your employer and it's insurance company to get adequate medical care and income to live on.

Simply telling your employer that you were injured is not the same as filing a Workman's Compensation claim nor is filling out your employers injury form. To file for Worker's Compensation, you need a special claim form that is then sent into your state's Division of Workman's Compensation. While Social Security Disability is a federal program, Workers Compensation is regulated on the state level. In order to get through the steps in your state you either need to go on line and find out what the process is or hire an attorney who specializes in Workman's Compensation cases. Since you will have ongoing claims with RSD for treatment, it is best to hire an attorney who is familiar with the laws of your state and in helping you get the best care possible.

You will at some point be asked to go for an Independent Medical Examination (IME). This is a doctor, who represents your employer's Workman's Compensation insurance company. It is advisable that you take someone with you to this appointment to take notes during the examination. Bring a pain diary with you. If you have photos of the involved limb when it is in its worse flare, bring them. Bring along as much documentation to leave with the IME doctor as you can. This doctor works for the insurance company and not for you. In Appendix D you will find a list of articles that will help you explain RSD to either Social Security, Workman's Compensation , your lawyer and your judge.

At some point, you will have to appear in front of a judge in order to get your employer's Workman's Compensation Insurance to pay for the treatments that your doctor recommends. This is another situation where having an attorney can help you. The insurance companies have highly pain lawyers on their side. They want to pay as little as possible to you.

Whether it be filing for SSD or fling a Workman's Compensation Claim it is going to be a stressful time. Stress increases the pain of RSD by stimulating your sympathetic (fight or flight) response. Having friends/ family who understand RSD and are supportive of you is important at this time.

When searching for a lawyer, make sure that he/she has experience in either SSD or WC cases. Ask for references. Ask how many claims they have won for SSD and what the awards were for WC cases. Make sure that you provide them with background information on RSD. Print out articles or refer them to web sites on RSD. You can also check him/her out through the American Bar Association and the Better Business Bureau. You've got a lot riding on paperwork being filed correctly and in a timely fashion. You want to be sure that your lawyer has experience in the type of case that you have.

Personal Injury Law Suits Your injury may be the result of someone else's negligence such as a car accident. How your medical bills are paid for through auto insurance varies from state to state. In addition to your medical bills you most likely have lost of income and will want compensation for pain and suffering. Beware of advertisements that will hook you up with a doctor and a lawyer; the ones that end in "non–attorney spokesman". You will want to find a lawyer that specializes in personal injury. Ask for references. Ask how many lawsuits of this kind they have won. How many times have they been to trial? You can check them out the same way you would with a SSD or WC lawyer. Again be sure that they are knowledgable about RSD. If they aren't, educate them.

Just as with a WC insurance claim, the auto insurance company will want an independent medical exam. Take someone with you to take notes. They work for the insurance company and not for you. Bring a pain diary with you. If you have photos of the involved limb when it is in its worse flare, bring them. Bring along as much documentation to leave with the IME doctor as you can.

Continuing to Work You may want to or need to continue to work after your injury. Your employer must make reasonable accommodations to make it possible for you to do your job. This may mean a special chair, frequent breaks, or other alterations to your workplace. It is a federal law that if you have a disability, your employer much make reasonable accommodations. You can find information on the ADA law at: www.ada.gov/. When considering whether or not to continue working, keep in mind that stress increases the pain levels of those with CRPS. If your job is stressful, you may want to look for a position that is less stressful.

Chapter 5
GRIEVING

When we suffer a loss, such as the loss of our former life with the diagnosis of CRPS, we grieve that loss much like we grieve the death of a loved one. This grieving cycle is divided into five components that don't we don't necessarily go through in this exact order. We may feel one stage more than another and may not experience some of them all. It is helpful to look at them as a guide for your own grieving process to help you morn the life that you had before RSD.

Denial and Isolation This is usually the first reaction to a diagnosis of CRPS. At first you can't believe that it is true. You become overwhelmed with emotions. You think that you are the only one that this has happened to or that it really isn't real. You stop going out with friends and family to avoid talking about your diagnosis. This is a defense mechanism that buffers the immediate shock. It carries you through the first wave of pain.

Anger As the masking effects of denial and isolation wear off, it is normal to become angry; "why me?" "what did I do to deserve this?. The intense emotion that we feel is deflected and redirected as anger.

Bargaining The normal reaction to feelings of helplessness and venerability is to try to regain control. "If only I'd sought medical attention sooner…" "If only I'd gotten a second opinion…" "if only I hadn't done (whatever it is that caused your injury)…"

Depression Depression is normal with a devastating diagnosis of CRPS. It is important for you to seek help from a psychologist/psychiatrist who has experience in working with chronic pain patients. Although depression does not cause CRPS, it can increase your pain. Do not let anyone tell you that the pain is all in your head. The pain is real and it can then lead to depression. When you are sad and emotional, it sends your sympathetics (your fight or flight) into over drive. This can make your pain worse. It is important to talk about how you are feeling, to know that you are not alone. In addition to working with a therapist, this is where support groups can come into play as they help you to realize that you are not alone in this. There are many medications to treat depression and your psychiatrist will make recommendations. Some antidepressants can serve a dual purpose. Effexor, for example, is an NMDA receptor antagonist (it blocks a nerve receptor that conducts pain impulses) and can actually help with pain.

Acceptance Acceptance of the diagnosis of CRPS does not mean you are giving up. It simply means that you need to work out a new normal for yourself. You still need to fight for the right treatment for yourself. Making informed decisions about your health care is important and empowering. Once that you've accepted CRPS, you are free to use informed consent to find the right treatment.

Often things like anniversaries of your injury or diagnosis, holidays or family functions can send you backwards in this process. This too is normal as long as you don't get stuck there. Grieving is a fluid process that you work through on an ongoing basis.

Getting involved in activities that you can do, meeting others with CRPS, and working out a new normal for your life. These things will help you to cope better with the diagnosis of CRPS. It's a process of trial and error as you learn what aggravates you pain and what doesn't. You will learn to pace yourself, to do one thing at a time rather than all at once. Knowledge is empowering, so learn everything that you can about this disease.

It is important to have a good support system. You may find that old friends fade away either because they don't know what to say or do or because they are sick of hearing about your CRPS. These people were never really true friends. Since getting CRPS, most of my old friends are no longer friends but I have made new friends who only know me as I am now and accept me for who I am.

It is possible for positive things to come from this diagnosis. I was once asked to write a list of positive things that have come from my CRPS diagnosis. Here is what I wrote:

I have met so many special people that I would have never met had I not had CRPS:

* I know who my real friends are

*I am more in tune with my body

*I have more tolerance for others

*I am my best advocate

*I know what is most important in life

*I know the importance of family

*I am now not afraid to ask for help when I need it

*I am a stronger person

*I am a nurse.

I had an AS in nursing but graduated from with my bachelor's degree just ten months before having the car accident that caused my CRPS. I continued to work but changed my the type of nursing that I did from direct nursing care to more of an administrative type of nursing. I worked with insurance companies getting nursing approved for chronically ill children whose parents needed to have help in order to keep their children at home. At that time in Pennsylvania, Medicaid was assigned to these chronically ill children. I had to write a waiver for Medicaid describing why the child needs nursing care. I became very good at it. Many people with CRPS who have had to stop working, like I have, feel useless and lack a purpose. Well I have found my niche. Most of us are being denied the treatments that our doctors have ordered to treat our CRPS or medications that we need. Because I spent the first five years struggling to keep working with my CRPS and learned the art of fighting insurance companies, not only has it benefited me in my battles with the health insurance companies; but I am able to offer my knowledge to others. Most of us have limited incomes such as Social Security Disability or Workman's Compensation payments. Being able to help others with CRPS by helping them fight their insurance battles gives me a sense of purpose again. It also helps them get the treatments and/or medications that they need and may not be able to win those battles themselves.

Take a minute and write down all of the positive things that CRPS has brought into your life. Concentrate on those things and not the negative things that RSD has brought to your life.

One sad fact is that there is a very high suicide rate among those who have CRPS If you have any thoughts of suicide, it is important to seek help immediately. See Appendix E for the names and phone numbers of suicide hot lines where you can talk to someone 24/7.

CHAPTER 6
FEELINGS

Often the person with RSD feels very alone. You are sure that there is no one else who experiences what you going through. Many people benefit from a support group wether it be an on line support group or a local social group of people with CRPS who get together once a month. In choosing a support group, you want to be sure that it is truly a supportive group and not a bitching session. There are several CRPS groups on Facebook, Yahoo, Neuro-talk, and Google. Check them out and find out which one works best for you.

RSDSA.org has a list of support groups in different parts of the country. They are a great resource for all sorts of information including the names of local support groups. AmericanRSDHope.org is another great resource. They offer mentors to newly diagnosed people with RSD. They also have a list of support groups.

It is important to know that you aren't alone. The more information that you can gather about CRPS the better your treatment choices will be and the more self confident you will feel in dealing with doctors, therapists as well as friends and families.

There is a letter in by Keith Orsini of RSDHope that describes what it is like to have CRPS. I enclosed it in my Christmas cards early on in my battle with CRPS to help people that were close to me to understand the disease and how it affected me. If you plan on using this, please be sure to give credit to the author.

"Letter To Families & Friends of CRPS Patients

written by Keith Orsini
March 2005

(For those of you who don't have RSD/CRPS but suffer from any other form of chronic pain (CP) you could probably substitute your disease everywhere you see the letters RSD in this article and share it with your families as well, and of course RSD has since been changed to CRPS)

Dear Loved Ones;

The other day a friend of mine asked me if I would share with her loved ones the experience of being an CRPS patient; what we go through on a daily basis, the struggles we face, and the importance of medications and therapy in our lives. I thought the best way to do this was to share what a typical day in the life of an CRPS patient was like. I myself have had CRPS since 1974, over thirty years now. I also have Degenerative Disc Disease, Failed Back Syndrome, Ulnar Nerve Entrapment, CFID'S, and Fibromyalgia so Chronic Pain (CP) and I are old friends. I first developed RSD when I was 14 years old.

Over the last 38+ years I have talked to tens of thousands of CRPS and other CP patients of all ages and we all experience pretty much the same things with some minor differences. As an example, for those who do care but are unsure what a typical day is for us, I will try to explain. Please don't take this letter as mean-spirited in any way. I know some of it may be hard to read, to actually see some of the words in print, but it is not an attack. Your loved ones just want their voices heard.

Over the years I have actually had people tell me, "Gee, it must be nice to get SSDisability, not have to work and just sit home all day". If I thought they were really interested in a reply to that ridiculous statement I would tell them that having CRPS and/or other CP Diseases, however severely you have it, is much more work than any full-time job! Plus, we don't get to call in sick, get vacation days, and our work day is 24 hours long, 7 days a week!

Now understand that quite a few CRPS and CP patients have other diseases as well, such as Fibromyalgia, Spinal Stenosis etc., and that some have it in one limb while for others it has spread to other areas; some have less movement while others have quite a bit; some take only a few medications, others quite a lot. I myself used to take a little over a total of 20 pills a day (thankfully a lot less today). Contrary to some people's opinions taking a pile of medications does not make us ""druggies". A druggie may be someone's idea of a person who takes drugs for recreation. A pain patient is someone who takes medication because he/she has no choice and who probably cannot fathom someone who takes narcotics for "fun and/or recreation"!

There are patients who use different types of machines, have Spinal Column Stimulators, or Pumps installed in their bodies in an attempt to reduce their pain. Some deal with the wheelchair issue as well. Most patients, the lucky ones at least, also do some form of physical therapy such as swimming, weights, or massage, or walking to help them continue to be able to do the basics of life and using their hands, feet, and arms.

First, let's start with the sleep patterns, or lack-of-sleep patterns to be more accurate. Unlike "normal" people, CP patients are prone to insomnia and do not reach REM sleep; this is the healing sleep our bodies need each day. We either wake often or are in a drug induced sleep. When we do wake, it is often physically painful to actually get up and out of bed. So, why don't we sleep? It is because CRPS cause changes to the Limbic System of the brain. The limbic system is that part of the brain that controls insomnia, short-term memory, concentration, irritability, ability to find the right word when speaking, and much more.

We start our day with medications of course. The first of many such times per day. To "look fine" we take 10 to 30 or more pills a day for various symptoms. Then there are the side effects of those medications to deal with; upset stomach, drowsiness, diarrhea, constipation, headaches, and many others. Many of us also have to fight the "Dry-Eye Syndrome" and must use eye drops two or more times per day, or dry mouth issues, or both. Understand that these pills do not take all of the pain away. They just enable us to get up, move around, and have some semblance of a "normal" life; they simply allow us to function. Then many of us head to Physical Therapy such as pool exercise, range of motion therapy, massage therapy, and even acupuncture. For the patients for whom these things work, they are lifesavers. Like the medications they allow us to function, to be a part of our families, to enjoy part of each day, and for some they actually give us a reason to get up in the morning. The lucky ones get out and walk and a few may even get out and work part-time or volunteer a few hours/days a week. The more we can do, the better it is for us, mentally and physically.

These aren't luxuries but necessities for those of us. We do them as much as our bodies can handle them, even pushing ourselves beyond our pain levels, knowing we will pay a pain-toll later. Because the alternative is to sit and do nothing, letting our bodies get worse and our minds waste away. Unfortunately many people see us during these times and see us as "normal" because our pain is invisible. What they can't see is the pain, mental and physical, we are pushing down just to be there as well as the price we will be paying later that day and night. Understand, I am not playing a pity card. I am just trying to share what our day is like. It might help you understand why we try to do thing in spurts, an hour or two at a time.

There can be month's, even years, when the allodynia is too high to do even these simple things. (Allodynia is when even the lightest touches or sounds cause extreme pain.) Maybe the person sitting next to you at dinner touches your RSD arm, or your foot gets accidentally kicked at the pew at Church, or your leg gets bumped into at school; all these things seem harmless to the average person and they may not understand how they could ever cause pain to an CRPS patient, but trust me, they can and do. Some people can even have a light breeze cause them excruciating pain.

I know what you are thinking, "that is crazy". No. That

is CRPS. If you think it's crazy, and I am telling you from a personal knowledge background, think how a patient who knows nothing about the disease feels when they start forgetting things, especially when their pain is high? Or when the slightest touch, even the caress of a loved one, the kiss from a spouse, the touch of the sheet on the foot, the tightness of a sock, sometimes even the very breeze itself blowing over the body, can cause such pain to the patient it will bring tears to their eyes. Think of the confusion and terror that brings into their lives.

And when their friend and loved ones sit there, makes fun of them, and disbelieves them when they try to explain how it causes pain, well, that hurts them even more. When a disconnected Doctor doesn't believe you that is bad enough but when a loved one doesn't believe you it hurts almost as much as the pain. And let me set the record straight here on the pain, there is no pain like the pain of RSD/CRPS. That isn't just from a patient or an advocate, it is documented. CRPS pain is ranked higher than any other form of chronic pain known today.

CRPS is ranked on the McGill Pain Index as the MOST PAINFUL FORM OF CHRONIC PAIN THAT EXISTS TODAY! To put that in perspective, you can visit a page we have on the website that shows some other diseases/conditions and their rankings. (click on the link above and scroll down to the index). As you can see on the scale, Arthritis pain is ranked about a 18, Cancer pain a 24, Chronic Back Pain a 26, and then CRPS is ranked a whopping 42!

The only thing close to CRPS pain is the amputation of

a finger and that is quick, CRPS is 24 hours a day, 7 days a week. Does that bring it home to you? It is a pain like no other. When people ask me to describe it to them the best I can do is say "Imagine you had CRPS in your hand and arm. Empty the blood from your blood vessels in your hand and arm, then refill them with lighter fluid and light them on fire. Keep them lit 24 hours a day, 7 days a week." Let that sink in for a moment. "Now imagine no else can see the flames or will believe that you are in pain no matter what you say". That is what CRPS feels like.

Whether we patients are walking for therapy, which I assure you is as painful as it is necessary, or doing things that remind us we are alive there is always a price to pay in extra pain directly afterwards, or even the next day or week. CRPS patients are cognizant of that every day. While the average person can sit there and tell us "Go ahead and enjoy the day, you can't let your pain control your life!"

What they don't realize is that we are controlling our pain and not the other way around. We control our pain by controlling what we do. What do I mean by doing things to remind us we are alive? When we spend a few hours tending the garden, spending time with our children, volunteering and trying to better our community, playing with our pets, going to a movie, grocery shopping, running errands, attending a family gathering, or even just going to church. Things that make us feel normal, if only for a few hours.

Unfortunately some people who see you during these "good times" believe that is how you are the entire day. What they don't see is the pain you experienced that night and/or the next day because of what you did. Nor do they take into account all the medications you took before or afterwards to enable you to do those things, nor the fact that you probably had to spend a great deal more time resting afterwards. The same is true for patients who go to the computer to get support from others with CRPS through cyberpals, listservs or websites. Many non-patients do not understand, that it is the time we spend there that keeps us going each day . It informs us of new procedures or medications and educates not only ourselves but also our loved ones and sometimes even our Doctors about how to cope/treat CRPS. For most of us it is our lifeline, not our toy. The time we spend on the computer is absolutely necessary to our general well-being for it is there that we can talk with others who truly understand what we deal with every day and every minute.

Many of us have to sneak in a nap in the afternoon to rest our bodies, especially those of us who also struggle with Fibromyalgia in addition to the CRPS. One of the problems this leads to is when our loved ones try to do something nice for us and plan a whole days activities. Sometimes it may be just too much for us. Because of this disease, you have to change your whole way of thinking to include doing things in moderation. For many people that means scheduling things in the morning when we are at our strongest and our pain is at its lowest. For others, it is much easier to do something in the late morning or early afternoon but typically by early evening we are done for the day. You also have to factor in your physical therapy and Doctor appointments as sometimes these things will wear us out for the entire day.

Another strange symptom that has to be factored into our daily lives is that many are bothered by vibrations and/or noise, and for a small percentage, it can actually make the pain skyrocket! A simple ride in the car over a bumpy road can cause a spike in pain. Due to the noise and vibrations causing me extra pain, for instance, there are a lot of things I cannot do, places I cannot go, and again, I am just one example of many out there. These are places most people take for granted and may wonder why we are not there. They may think we are shutting ourselves off by not going, places like my Church where the organ music can be very painful, my Masonic Meetings, going out with friends, etc. If there are a lot of people making noise, even if it is simply singing or clapping, a baby crying, it can cause our pain to spike. Visits sometimes have to be cut short due to all the regular noise that is typically generated, or we just have to go off to another room; and don't even start on things like thunderstorms, whew!

Imagine saying to your boss, "Sir, I have to go home, the thunder is causing me great pain and the strong wind blowing is hurting me as well." Oh yeah, they would love that. Sorry I can't come to your birthday party because there will be too many people having fun and enjoying themselves and making noise. Yeah, that makes sense, especially to my 10 year old niece. I can only imagine the restrictions parents with kids have to place on their children so as not to hurt their CRPS limbs, after all kids will be kids. I was lucky when I was a teen with CRPS because, despite many a day spent wearing dark glasses due to the pain of the bright sunlight or the days when the pain of my RSD made the ordinary things extremely difficult, my friends were always there. So many teens I talk to on our RSDHope Teen Corner aren't as lucky. They have schoolmates who take pleasure in pushing them in the hallway to see them fall on their bad leg, or purposefully hit their CRPS arm. Why, even their own siblings hurt them or taunt them about their CRPS, as if it is something they have a choice in. Who would choose CRPS? Do they think if we just decide to smile it will go away? It would even be a little more understandable if it were just the kids. Unfortunately it isn't, as many of you personally know.

I have heard so many stories from our teens with CRPS/CP whose siblings, Aunts, Uncles, even parents, who tell them they need to "Just get over it, deal with it, move on already". Great advice from the uneducated and seemingly uncaring. Instead of saying things like that, why not read up on the disease, go to the websites like ours, see what the truth is regarding using the limbs, talk with the Doctor about it if you really care that much about their well-being. You don't know how much it would mean to the patient if you took just an hour here and there to do that.

The bottom line here and the points I have tried to get across are that;
When you suffer from chronic pain, you have to constantly think about how, whatever you are going to do that day, will affect your disease and your pain level.

Being in chronic pain is a full-time job.

One with no vacations, terrible benefits, and no way to

quit.

CRPS is the most painful form of chronic pain that exists today and currently there is no cure.

Chronic pain affects the entire family, not just the patient.

Chronic pain is an invisible disability. Even other pain patients will sometimes forget that they cannot see YOUR pain and make assumptions based on what they can visibly see.

A chronic pain patient may have a good hour or even many good hours a day where they can "appear normal" to everyone else but most don't realize the price that is paid before and after.

The positive involvement of their loved ones means the world to the chronic pain patient.

I am still surprised at the number of fellow pain patients who forget that not everyone with CRPS, and/ or other forms of chronic pain, show outward signs of it ALL the time, so it is understandable when our loved ones forget. Never assume you know someone else's whole story at a glance. I spent a few years being stuck in bed unable to walk. I spent well over a year being confined to a wheelchair (which they told me to buy not rent) and then had to learn how to walk again. That was the second time in my life I have had to do that, despite being told by Drs that I may not ever be able to walk again. Good thing I am stubborn.

I remember one year where the only time I was able to

leave my room was to go to physical therapy five days a week. I have spent many years having to use a cane to go even ten feet and despite this, I still have people who don't know anything about my past struggles, even some who are fellow CRPS patients, email me and tell me I have no idea what it is like to be stuck in a chair or be unable to walk! That I don't have it as tough as they do. Yes, this is a very difficult disease and every case is a little different but don't let others convince you, not even your Drs, that your case is so unique, "the worst case they have ever seen", that it makes you throw in the towel and just give up. FIGHT!

I am blessed in that currently, I am doing better than many other years. That doesn't mean I am "cured". I take my pills each day. I have to do my physical therapy every day. I have to walk every day. Nearly every afternoon is spent having to lie down because of exhaustion, partly due to the CRPS and partly due to the CFIDS and Fibromyalgia, in combination with the medications. Evenings, my pain escalates such that I rarely go out. But I am not complaining. I have been much worse in my life and I never forget it for a minute. But NEVER compare your pain to someone else's. It is a lose–lose situation. It hurts you both. Instead encourage one another and support your fellow pain patients! We all deal with pain in different ways and we all have different levels of tolerance.

Our medications, our therapies, and our friends are what get us through each day. The value of none of these things can be minimized. Not just for the physiological changes that they bring to our body but for the psychological ones as well. That doesn't mean our lives end, they just change. And CRPS/CP patients require tools to make those changes possible. Tools that include medication, various therapies, exercise, diet changes, and lots of familial support. You can be a positive part of it or you can be a hindrance, it is totally up to you.

Now some may view this as being obsessed with the disease, that we think of nothing else but our disease, our pain, that we are too focused on it and that is why we are so depressed, so sad, we hurt so much. Gee, you mean if I didn't think about it so much I wouldn't hurt so much? Hmm, let me give that a try. dum – dum – de – dum – de – dum dum dumb dumb dumb. Nope, didn't work. Shocking.

No, seriously, the fact is that for us, CRPS/CP is a major part of our life. It has to be factored into every decision we make, if it isn't we will pay for it later, as will our loved ones. My family and I often worry that our friends will get tired of our talking about CP too often. After all, not only have I had it for years but most of our family is involved in running this organization and getting the word out about this disease. Many times we have to force ourselves to take a break from CRPS talk for a day. But then we think it is no different than if we had cancer, MS, or MD, (which some of us have). People are just used to hearing those words more. Yes, we will lose friends along the way, that is inevitable But we will also gain some new wonderfully supportive friends and they will be amazing, true friends who will be in it for the long haul.

I cannot tell you all the incredible people from all over the world I have met in our journey, with whom I have become fast friends. Some I see often and some I see only at our National Conferences on Pain yet it is as if I saw them just yesterday; many I talk to only on-line and I know them best of all. These are amazing people who have overcome obstacles you wouldn't believe and yet still come out on top. And you know what? They could care less that I have CRPS. So now that YOU know what it is all about ... which type of friend are you? I hope this has helped you better understand a day in the life of an CRPS/CP patient and that you didn't take it as a slap in the face or something hurled at you but as a teaching tool. Sometimes we have to be forced to confront things in our lives in a harsh manner in order to accept that they are real; both the patient and the loved one in the case of the chronic pain patient. Thanks for listening/reading.

Peace, Keith Orsini
American RSDHope

On behalf of Chronic Pain patients everywhere, thank you for taking the time to read this. It means a great deal to them that you would take the time to do this and just because they asked you to read this does not always mean they feel they have a problem with you necessarily, they just wanted you to have a better idea about what they have to deal with. They NEED you in their life; they WANT you beside them in this struggle. They know they can do it; they can beat this with YOUR help.

copyright March/2005-2012

Please feel free to share this article with others, we just ask that you respect and include the copyright and author information."

CHAPTER 7
FINDING WAYS TO COPE

Finding your new normal Once you have accepted your diagnosis of CRPS, finding a "new normal" is the next step. Some of the things you loved to do before getting CRPS may no longer be possible. Some of your friends and family members may not understand what you are going through and may fade away. This can be very difficult. Try to educate the people who you are close to you. The ones who can't make the adjustment weren't really your friends anyway. If you are no longer working then you may feel isolated from the rest of the world.

The first thing that you need to figure out is what things increase your pain and what things help your pain. You need to learn to pace yourself so that you can minimize your pain. When I'm considering an activity, I try to be sure that it is not something that will cause my CRPS to flare. It comes down to are the negative side effects of increased pain worth the importance of the task. Some times your answer will be no and you will turn down an invitation or not do something that you used to love doing. Other times, the task is important enough that it is worth a few days of increased pain.

You may feel very isolated and alone. If you are not working out in the world with other people then you don't want to stay in the house feeling sorry for yourself. Making friends with others with chronic pain through support groups and on line groups may make you feel less isolated. Making a regular date to go out and do something that you enjoy will help you feel less isolated. Just getting out of the house to do something other than go to another doctor's appointment or test is important. If your CRPS doesn't affect your feet or legs, plan on a daily walk. If walking is too painful, utilize what ever adaptive equipment you can use to get out. I have CRPS in my foot and at the young age of 38, I found myself using a wheelchair just to be able to get out with my husband and children. At first it was humiliating, but then I realized it was either use a wheelchair, miss out on the activities or over do things and increase my pain. I opted for the wheelchair. Fortunately, I was able to get my doctor to write an order for it and my insurance covered it. This is not always the case. Check with local medical supply companies to see if they have used wheelchairs to purchase. If that is too much of an expense, check out local charities such as Goodwill to see if they have any donated ones.

It is important to find a hobby that you are able to do without increased pain. For me, it was scrapbooking. Anyone that I knew who was getting married or having a baby, I would give them a home made certificate for a scrapbook of the event. I also love photography so in many instances, I would offer to take the photos as well. Distraction is a wonderful thing to help you deal with pain. Anything that takes your mind off of the pain is wonderful. Others enjoy making jewelry, painting or sewing.

Sleep and coping mechanisms Another problem that most of us deal with is insomnia. Chronic pain often makes it difficult to sleep. Sleep is crucial. Sleep deprivation is used as a for of torture. For those of us with chronic pain, sleep is even more important. Sleep restores your energy levels and helps combat fatigue. Eventually lack of sleep reduces your immune system making your more susceptible to other illnesses. Additionally, because of the some of the medications that we take, we are more prone to nightmares. These can further disturb normal sleep patterns. Our ability to cope with our chronic pain is also disrupted by lack of proper sleep.

Stages of sleep There are definite states of sleep. The first stage of sleep is the hypnogogic state, as you are just dragnet off to sleep. The next period, REM (Rapid Eye Movement) sleep is where dreams happen. During REM sleep, you lose muscle tone. During this phase your body can not move. You can't be dreaming and tossing and turning at the same time.

There are different types of sleep disturbance. Whenever your pain is increased, you will have more difficulty falling asleep. There are two basic types of sleep disturbance; alpha-delta anomaly and insomnia. In alpha-delta sleep disturbance, the alpha waves that are usually happening during your waking hours intrude into your sleeping hours. Higher levers of these alpha waves during sleep will make you more sensitive to pain. Insomnia, on the other hand, means that you just can't sleep right. Stress is the major cause of insomnia. Insomnia falls into three categories; onset insomnia, maintenance insomnia and early a.m. insomnia. In onset insomnia, you have difficulty falling asleep. Maintenance insomnia finds you waking up in the middle of the night while early a.m. insomnia is where you wake up too early and are not able to fall back to sleep.

Lack of sleep magnifies your pain, depression and your ability to adapt to your new life. There are different tricks to getting to sleep. Journaling not only helps to make you drowsy but it is an important record of your daily pain that can be beneficial for your treatment or a court case. It helps to remove stress from your body and get a better nights sleep. Meditation before bedtime is another way to relax your body and mind. Turning down the lights in the hour before you go to sleep can help you nod off to sleep. Having a regular sleep schedule is important. Have a set time that you go to bed each night and don't deviate from it by going to bed too early or two late. Daytime napping can also interfere with your sleep at night. Be sure to keep all electronics out of your bedroom. The bedroom should be a place for sleep and not for going on line, watching TV, cell phone use or other stimulating activities. The room should be dark and quiet. White noise machines can be helpful to lull you to sleep.

If you have done all of these things and you are still having disturbed sleep, it may be time to consult a sleep specialist. They may ask you to do a sleep study. This is where you are in a special hospital room from about 8:30 p.m. until 7:00 a.m. You are hooked up to a EEG (measures your brainwaves), heart monitor, oxygen saturation monitor, and respiratory monitor. There are cameras observing your sleep in addition to the monitors recording your vital signs as your sleep. From this test, they can be sure that you aren't having apnea (the cessation of breathing) during your sleep as well as monitoring the depth of your sleep using the EEG recording. Following the sleep study, you may be prescribed a CPAP (continuous positive airway pressure) machine to help with any sleep apnea that you might have. The doctor may also prescribe a sleep aide to help you either fall asleep, or stay asleep.

When your pain is at its worse there are things that you can do to help you cope. Many pain management offices offer Biofeedback. Biofeedback is a way to train your brain to change the pain signals. You are hooked up to a machine that measures your heart rate and blood pressure. You learn to relax and make your body react the way that you want it to do. Guided imagery is another way of coping with chronic pain. There are CDs that help talk you into a state of relaxation through guided imagery. Taking a warm Epsom Salts soak can also help you to relax and sooth the pain. When your body is tense, the pain intensifies. By finding a way to relax whether it be through meditation, yoga, guided imagery or biofeedback; you can increase your ability to cope with chronic pain by having an arsenal of tools at your disposal.

CHAPTER 8
FACT OR FICTION

There is a lot of misinformation about RSD/CRPS. Many health care professionals have misconceptions about RSD and others do not even recognize the term CRPS. Here are some common misconceptions:

There is no such thing as RSD; it's all in your head: I can't tell you how many times that I have heard this. It is not all in your head. CRPS is a physiologic change in the body. There are physical changes that can't be denied. There physical changes were discussed previously. Anyone who says that CRPS is all in your head has no idea what they are talking about and they should not be treating someone with CRPS.

Use ice: Ice should never be used by someone with CRPS. Even though the person with CRPS feels burning pain, ice is one of the worst things that you can do to relieve your pain. Normally during physical therapy for an injury they alternate ice and heat. The application of ice results in stimulation of the sympathetic system. Secondary constriction of the superficial sympathetic vasoconstrictors occurs. Heat, on the other hand, results in the dilatation of superficial blood vessels and the relaxation of the vasoconstrictor activity of the sympathetic nervous system. In CRPS, the goal is to warm the extremity which is already cooler than the rest of the body, to dilate the superficial blood vessels and to slow down the simultaneous inflammation. The goal is to increase circulation in the deep structures of the extremities. Heat will increase circulation and slow down inflammation whereas cold decreases circulation and increases the inflammatory response. Ice has no place in the treatment of the chronic pain of CRPS.

CRPS/RSD does not spread: It sure can! CRPS is not usually limited to one part of an extremity or even just one extremity. The first areas to be affected are the pathways of the sympathetic nerves between the injured extremity and the spinal cord. This results in inflammation and irritation of the nerves from that extremity to the spinal cord.   The next area of CRPS involvement is the spinal cord. This is manifested by movement disorders, muscle spasms, and weakness of the extremity. CRPS moves up the extremity as more sympathetic nerves between the injury and the spinal cord are involved. It can cross over to the opposite side where the person with CRPS has mirroring symptoms on the opposite side from the original injury.   The sympathetic system is complex, bilateral and diffuse. CRPS is complex, bilateral and diffuse in its spread. Some people have little CRPS spread while others have full body spread. The degree to which CRPS spreads varies from person to person.

Depression is causing your pain; This is an example of which came first, the chicken or the egg. For people with CRPS, the pain comes first. Being in pain all of the time along with the changes that it makes in your life, your relationships with others, your ability to work all cause depression. It is important for people with RSD to seek out professional help from a psychiatrist or psychologist who specializes in chronic pain. Chronic pain can be overwhelming and it is important to find the right therapist to help you manage your depression. Anger, frustration and depression are all common feelings that accompany CRPS. "Why me?", "What did I do to deserve this?" are common feelings from people with CRPS. They are normal feelings. It is how you manage these feelings that is important. The person with RSD is grieving for the life that they had prior to their CRPS. They are morning lost relationships, the loss of a career, and changes in the way that they perceive themselves. Of course you are going to be depressed when on top of non-stop pain, you have all of these other changes in your life. Anniversaries, holidays and other triggers may cause you to regress in your process through the grieving cycle. Little set backs are normal. It is important that you discuss these set backs with your mental health professional. Antidepressants are common in treatment of the depression that accompany CRPS. The suicide rates among those with CRPS is high. This is one of many reasons why it is important to seek help from either a psychiatrist or psychologist who is familiar with chronic pain.

With physical therapy no pain no gain is the rule: This is absolutely false. The goal of physical therapy, occupational therapy and aqua therapy are to help the person with CRPS get moving. The purpose is to do so without increasing pain. There are instances where the phrase "no pain, no gain" are true as when athletes are training. With CRPS, it does not apply. Therapeutic aqua therapy where you are moving in warm water can be a very effective way to keep moving with a positive effect. The warm water is soothing to most and the buoyancy takes your weight off of joints that may be painful. The goal of therapy is to help elevate pain by helping the RSeDr to keep their limbs moving so that they don't stiffen up or lock up which causes additional pain. The goal of therapy is not to inflict pain.

CRPS can not go into remission: When CRPS is diagnosed within the first three to six months, the disease can go into remission in some patients provided that they are treated appropriately. There should not be excessive bed rest, excessive exercise, ice application, surgery, sympathectomy or strong narcotic treatment.   CRPS will stay with a patient the rest of their life if they are: misdiagnosed or diagnosis is delayed two years or longer, if there is additional trauma due to surgery, and treatment that involves sympathectomy, amputation of the insertion of a needle into the area of CRPS for blocks or other purposes. Often when remission is achieved, another simple injury will bring it back. At this time, there is no cure for CRPS.

CHAPTER 9
REMISSION: WHAT IT IS AND HOW DOES IT OCCUR

What is remission? Remission occurs when all of the CRPS symptoms disappear after treatment. You might ask, if my symptoms are gone aren't I cured? In most people who experience remission, it is short lived. Another injury, surgery, and stress can all bring the symptoms back. The effect of treatments that can lead to remission are often short lived.

In a study, RSDSA (Reflex Sympathetic Dystrophy Syndrome Association) surveyed a survey when first diagnosed with CRPS. Of those who then went on to fill out a second survey 88.3% (264 of 299 completing both surveys) were female and 44.8% (134 of 299 completing both surveys) were between the ages of 45 and 55 years of age. Remission was reported by 16.5% (44 of 99 patients taking both surveys). Patients who reported relief from sympathetic blocks were more likely to experience remission. The type and location of their injury, demographics, time of diagnosis and duration of systems were not statistically significant predictors of reemission. Of those who experienced remission 84.1% (37 of the 44) had recurrence of their CRPS symptoms. The length of remission varied from 0 to 20 years with a mean of 2.01 years. Based on this study, it appears that sympathetically maintained symptoms are more likely to achieve remission. That remission is often transient, with most having a recurrence of symptoms. (RDSA.org February 1999)

Sympathetically maintained pain is pain that exist independently in that there is no injury to nerve tissue. After an injury to the soft tissue or bone, the pain persists after the injury has healed. The pain is disproportionate to the original injury and persists after the injury has healed. The sympathetic nervous system maintains the pain as opposed to pain associated with a direct injury to nerve tissue.

In a study done by Drs Rohr, Schwartzman, Ploppa, and Altimeter, Ketamine and remission were documented on a patient who presented with rapid progressing contiguous spread of CRPS. Standard medication and interventional therapy (blocks, epidurals, etc.) given successively failed to halt the spread of CRPS from the wrist to the entire right arm. The subjects pain was unmanageable with all standard therapy. As a last treatment option, the patient was transferred to the intensive care unit and treated on a compassionate care basis with anesthetic doses (anesthetic doses means a dose high enough to put you to sleep) of ketamine in gradually increasing doses of 3 – 5 mg per kilogram of weight per hour along with midazolam for a period of 5 days.

On the second day of the ketamine induced sleep, edema and discoloration began to resolve. An increase in spontaneous movement was noted. On day 6, symptoms completely resolved and the infusions were tapered. The patient woke up completely pain free and remained so for 8 years. This intensive care procedure has very serious risks but in this case, no severe complications occurred. The psychiatric effects were managed with the continued use of midazolam over the month following the initial treatment. (Pain Practice 2007 Jun; 7(2);147–50)

In a larger study published by Pain Medicine (2007) by Drs. Kiefer, Rohr, Ploppa, Dietrich, Grothusen, Koala, Altimeter, Unerl, and Schwartzman the looked at a larger number of patients with CRPS who had failed all other therapies. In this study 20 CRPS patients, who had not responded to standard treatments received ketamine in anethesetic dosages, along with other medications to prevent hallucinations, over five days. The criteria measured were pain relief, effect on movement disorder, quality of life and ability to work at baseline and up to 6 months following treatment. According to this study, low dose ketamine has been successful in patients with early localized pain but not in patients with advanced CRPS. Ketamine's analgesic potency and duration of affect in neuropathic pain are directly dose-dependent.

The results were significant pain relief was observed at 1, 3, and 6 months following the treatment. Complete remission for CRPS was observed at 1 month in all patients, at 3 months in 17 of the 20 patients, and at 6 months in 16 of the 20 patients. If relapse occurred, significant pain relief was still attained at 3 and 6 months. Quality of life, the associated movement disorder and the ability to work were significantly improved in the majority of patients at 3 and 6 months. The link to this study in is Appendix G along with other research studies. I was one of these 20 patients described in this study. You can read more about it in Chapter 13 where I tell my CRPS story.

At the time of the writing of this book, Ketamine given at anesthetic dosages (also referred to as a Ketamine Coma) is not available. Between 2001 and 2008, it was done in Germany. It was also offered in Monterrey Mexico until 2011. When the two studies were completed, the treatment was no longer offered. High dose Ketamine that is not anesthetic is offered by several physicians around the country. They have demonstrated remission in some of their patients with follow up ketamine infusions at a lower dosage.

In conclusion; for patients with sympathetically maintained pain remission is possible with sympathetic blocks. For patients who are diagnosed early and have not experienced a spread of their pain, low dose ketamine infusions have produced remission in some patients. For patients with advance spread of their CRPS, remission has been documented with the treatment of anesthetic doses of Ketamine.

So what does this mean for you? Depending on what your symptoms are and how long you have had your CRPS symptoms, these studies may help you decide along with your physician, the appropriate treatment that offers you the best chance of remission. Long term remission as seen in the patient who had eight years of remission are rare. For most, remission comes and goes. Although your goal may be remission, psychologically it is important to keep in mind that at this time there is no cure for CRPS. It can be psychologically devastating to count on any given treatment putting you into remission only to find that it doesn't happen or if it does it's short lived. Being hopeful and upbeat about the treatment you are receiving is a good attitude. To count on any given treatment resulting in remission and it not happening can be devastating.

CHAPTER 10
CHILDREN AND RSD

In recent years there has been an increase in the reporting of CRPS in children and adolescents. As with adults, early diagnosis and treatment is crucial. Children are resilient and their bodies are still growing and developing. With early diagnosis with an aggressive treatment plan, children have a better chance of going into remission.

As in adults, girls are five times more likely to develop CRPS than their male counter part. The incidence increases markedly just before puberty. Female dancers, gymnasts, and those participating in other competitive athletics make up a high percentage of children with CRPS. Untreated, the symptoms can be chronic, spread to other parts of the body and become chronic. The severity of the pain and the disruption of the child's life can lead to depression and anxiety especially if it goes undiagnosed and untreated. Disability in the pediatric population is described in terms of days of school missed. In a study done at Boston College Children's Hospital the average RSD patient had missed 40 days of school. With treatment, the average days of school missed dropped to less than five days per year. Yet children with RSD may miss school due to treatment.

With the school age child, there are also the issues of integrating the child's education with their CRPS. is estimated that 2.2 million children ages 14 and younger are injured in school related activities. Children ages 10 – 14 account for 46% of the school related injuries. (www.safekids.org)

There was a study done at Children's Hospital of Philadelphia where they followed 103 children through an intensive exercise program that involved four hours of therapy per day for fourteen days at a specialized center. The initial resolution of symptoms occurred in 92% of the children in the study. Two years later 88% remained symptom free. The key with these children is that they were diagnosed promptly and referred to a pediatric pain program promptly. The severity of the disability was directly related to the delay in diagnosis and the delay in referral to a proper pain management physician. Being immobilized also dramatically reduced the chance of remission in these children.

CRPS is poorly understood by many physicians so how can we expect our schools to understand it. A child's pain may be ignored or even mocked. Only the child in pain knows how much it hurts and their limitations. It is important if your child has CRPS that you provide your child's school with information on CRPS. Arrange for a conference call between your child's teachers and pain management physician.

Section 504 of the Rehabilitation Act (Appendix F) prohibits discrimination against individuals with disabilities. A child with RSD has equal access to an education. It is important that the needs of each child be met through accommodations. Some accommodations that have helped students with RSD are described in the website rsdsa.org. They are:

* Because the slightest bump can cause lasting flare-ups of this very painful syndrome, every effort should be made to see that the child is not exposed to the bumping and jostling of school hallways.

* The student' desk in each classroom should be positioned away from traffic patterns to avoid inadvertent bumping.

 *Determine whether the student needs ergonomic seating/ adjustable desk.

* Designate another student as a helper who can carry the student's books/belongings during the day, help at lunch, and during the changing of classes.

 *Because students with RSD/CRPS in their upper extremity

may have difficulty writing, allow the student to tape record lectures, use a keyboard with a portable word processor, or use another student's notes.

*Given that RSD/CRPS symptoms can be exasperated by the cold, allow the student to bring a heating pad.

*Also, guidelines should be developed regarding whether the child should go outside for recess when it is excessively cold; care must be taken to see that the patient has adequate warm clothing, and is kept out of drafts.

*Allow students to have an extra set of books at home in addition to school.

*Permit the student to go to the nurse when needed (may be experiencing a pain flare-up).

* Permit the student to leave 5 minutes prior to the end of class to avoid the congested hallways.

*Let the student stretch or take breaks whenever needed.

*Confer with parents as to whether they wish the classmates to be aware of the syndrome.

 *If there is a dress code, the child may need to adapt cloth-ing due to sensitivity to clothing and increased sweating.

*Special accommodations may be necessary for school field trips, including transportation, medication disbursement, and lodging (if an overnight trip).

*Limiting Stress Because stress is a known cause of exacerbation of this syndrome, academic schedules and curricula may have to be modified, including:
 Schedule all classes on one level or provide student with key to the elevator.

*Implement flexible homework and make-up policies (homework and tests are a major cause of additional stress).

*If a student is unable to write, modify normal test taking, and allow additional time for tests.

*Reduce school time if necessary (students may be late due to pain flare-ups) and supplement with home-based instruction and tutoring.

*If mobility is impaired, credit the student's physical/ occupational therapy as the requirement for gym (if the school has a pool, allow the student to use the pool during gym).

*Arrange special transportation if traveling on a crowded, bumpy school bus is too difficult.

* For older students, provide a designated handicapped parking space.

*Arrange for the student to meet with the school counselor on a regular basis.

As a parent, you must be your child's fierce advocate. Their pain is real. The mechanism that generates it is still poorly understood. You, as the parent of a child with CRPS, must become an expert on CRPS. You need to gather information to educate your child's principal,teachers and classmates. Here are some ideas:

*When you come across some good information on CRPS, make multiple copies to distribute to the teachers, school nurse, administrator, family and friends.

*Keep communications open with your child's school. Be clear about what modifications need to be made in the classroom.

*Find a support group for parents of children with CRPS.

*Use the Internet to become as informed as possible.

*Take cues from your child as to whether they want to participate in a support group for children/teens.

*Children and teens are dealing with issues of independence in addition to dealing with CRPS. This makes parental intervention difficult to navigate.

Encourage your child to be involved with his/her own treatment. Encourage them to speak up to the healthcare professionals rather than speaking through you.
Keep a positive attitude.

It is difficult enough navigating through childhood and adolescence. They need all of the support that they can get to navigate through it with CRPS. Let your child know that you believe in him/her and understand that their pain is real. Let your child take the lead.

Under the Disabilities Education Act (IDEA) your child is entitled to an Individualized Education Plan (IEP). So what is an IEP and how to I make sure that my child gets one. An IEP is a specialized learning plan that is created by your child's educators and you. There is an IEP meeting where the participants identify your child's specialized educational needs. This is where you need to be sure that everyone understands your child's unique needs. Be prepared with printed material about CRPS, medical records documenting what makes the child's pain worse or better, and a premeditated list of accommodations that you feel needs to be made by the school in order for your child to experience the least pain and get the best education.

A list of goals will be apart of the IEP. There can be additional meetings after the original IEP is developed to refine these goals if they are not obtainable by your child. There is no limit to the number of IEP meetings that can take place to discuss your child's education. Don't be intimidated by school administrators, teachers, or school nurses. Do some research to be sure that you know your child's educational rights and be prepared to fight for them.

For more information on pediatric pain, contact
www.TCAPP.org

CHAPTER 11
Pregnancy and CRPS

CRPS can affect a woman's hormones, however it is possible for a woman with CRPS to become pregnant and carry her baby to term. A man with CRPS is also capable of having children. The difficulty that the woman faces in pregnancy with CRPS is the method of pain management that they will use during pregnancy.

Most medications used to treat neuropathic pain are medications such as seizure medications. These medications can cause birth defects in the fetus. It is in the best interest of the fetus that as little medication as possible be taken during pregnancy. The first step before choosing to have a child is to consult a neonatologist and a high risk obstetrician. The neonatologist should be familiar with the effects of medication on the fetus.

If the mother decides to get pregnant and continues to take opioids during her pregnancy, her baby will be born addicted to that medication. The baby will need to be detoxified from the medication. This means that the baby will need to be born in a hospital that has a neonatal intensive care unit (NICU). The baby will be given methadone. The methadone will be weaned as tolerated by the baby. In some cases, depending on dosage and frequency with which the mom took the opioids will determine how long the baby will need to remain in the neonatal intensive care unit (NICU).

There is very little literature about CPRS and pregnancy. In the literature that exists, the women with CRPS had a decrease in their CRPS symptoms during pregnancy. Any trauma can cause an increase of CRPS symptoms or spread of CRPS symptoms; therefore a traumatic vaginal delivery could in fact cause CRPS of the vagina. Quite often a cesarean delivery is performed under spinal anesthesia. The spinal anesthesia should be continued for at least twenty four hours after the surgery.

How do you decide if you should have a child with CRPS? Here are some things to consider. Can you tolerate being off all medications during the pregnancy? Will you be able to care for the child with your CRPS? This is a decision that you and your spouse should make together. It is likely that the father will have to take a more active role in childrearing due to the mother's CRPS.

CHAPTER 12
CRPS True Stories

My Journey With CRPS/RSD
By Nancy Renée Cotterman

In my case, my injury was caused by a complex fracture that occurred in a car accident. It was March 4, 1996, I had just stopped at a Wawa to pick up some milk on my way home. I was working as a pediatric nurse in a home care company. I was on my way home from a case in Philadelphia. It was close to 7:00 p.m. I had traveled that road many times before. As I crested a hill; I came towards the intersection. The light was green, so I proceeded through the intersection. Out of nowhere, a nineteen year old, on her way to a date, made a left turn into the left front of my car. I saw her car a split second before we collided. I hit the brake just as our cars collided. At that moment, I felt a sharp pain shoot from my right foot up my leg. My foot must have absorbed all of the energy of the impact. I knew at that point that I had broken something although I had never broken a bone before. I felt pain like I had never felt before. I have two children, who I gave birth to naturally and yet, I'd never felt pain like that before in my life.

Two people who had been in the cars behind me told me that I had to get out of my smoking car. I told them that I couldn't, that I couldn't walk. They helped me out of the car and helped me to the curb. I sat there in the cold, stunned and in pain. The driver of the other car was slightly hysterical but physically unharmed. She kept repeating, "I'm sorry, I'm so sorry".

I was on call for the home company that I worked for. The first thing that went through my mind is that I needed to get off call NOW! I knew that I needed to call the other nurse that I worked with and get her to take call. Then I needed to call home. Although we had call waiting; when you have two daughters, they don't always pick up. My 13 year old had her own line, so I tried her line. She answered. I told her to get her father. She started asking a bunch of questions. I was not in the mood for idle conversation, so I repeated "get your father". I told my husband Jim that I was only a couple of miles from Bryn Mawr Hospital and that I would most likely be taken there. I told him that I would confirm that when the ambulance came. We live about 40 minutes from the hospital so he didn't wait for that second phone call and started off for the hospital.

My foot was swelling and throbbing with pain. I had to take my shoe off. A paramedic, who was not on duty, stopped at the accident scene and splinted my foot and ankle. Before I could thank him, he was gone. Finally after sitting out in the cold for what seemed like forever, the ambulance came. They took me by ambulance to Bryn Mawr Hospital (the hospital where I had worked as a nurse for 5 years). I had ridden in the ambulance as a nurse, but never as a patient. I had worked in that very emergency room as a nurse, but never had I been in there as a patient. This was the beginning of my education on seeing the medical profession from the other side, the side of the patient. And what an education it would be.

As I said, I had never broken a bone in my life. When I did on the cool March evening, I really did it. In the ER, they took x-rays and gave me a shot of Demerol. That shot of Demerol didn't touch the pain. I was screaming. My husband had never heard me scream like that. When I had my daughters, I was controlled and relaxed. I was prepared for that. I was frightened and in horrible pain now. The police officer came into the exam room to question me. He said that the other driver had admitted fault but he wanted to hear my story any how. He said that she would be sited for failure to yield and not to worry.

The orthopedic resident enlisted my husband's help in putting on the plaster splint and ace wrap on my right foot....big mistake. You never ask a family member to assist in a procedure like that. I was still screaming. My husband started turning sheet white. The resident told him to hold my big toe. The next thing you know, Jim was down and hit his head on the bottom of an IV pole. They took Jim into the next room, hooked him up to an EKG monitor and gave him a tetanus shot. I was the one waiting in a wheelchair for him so that I could go home. I was release with a pair of crutches and a prescription for pain medication along with a very embarrassed husband. I was told to follow up with an orthopedist the next day. The on call orthopedist was someone who I knew and had worked with for 5 years at that hospital. His specialty was foot and ankle orthopedics so he is who I contacted in the morning. I crawled up my stairs, got into bed and spent a long night in pain at home. I was told to put ice on my foot; one twenty minutes then off twenty minutes to help with the pain and swelling.

I met with the orthopedist (Dr. E) the next day and he ordered a CT scan to be sure that the bones are in place. The CT scan showed at least eight fractures in the mid-foot that were not displaced but were crushed. He told me to keep my leg elevated and iced so that the swelling will go down and then I could be casted. So I laid in my bed, getting calls from work asking me for help while I was on pain medication and hoping that the swelling would go down so that I could get back to work.

Finally ten days later it was time to put on the cast. I immediately went back to work. In hindsight, that was a bad idea. I still didn't even have a car yet but got a ride to work with a coworker. Almost immediately, I had begun to have burning pain in my foot even before the cast went on. I was not allowed to put any weight on my foot at all for eight weeks which was very difficult because our office was on the second floor with no elevator and outdoor stairs. The hallway was too narrow to use crutches. I used a small office chair on wheels, rested my knee on it and rolled around the office. One day, the shoelace of my left shoe got twisted in the wheel of the chair. I couldn't reach the wheel so I had to call for help to get my shoelace out of the wheel. That gave everyone a huge laugh!

At the end of the eight weeks in the cast, the orthopedist put me into an equalizer boot. I began to tell him about the burning sensation in my foot. My foot was purplish blue in color. I'd never broken a bone before nor had I taken care of someone who had as I never worked on an orthopedic floor. He would say that it was a bad fracture, give it time. It told me it would take a year for the fractures to completely heal. I waited.

Eight more weeks passed and the orthopedist wanted me to start wearing a sneaker. I couldn't tolerate putting my foot into a sneaker. The burning in my foot was getting worse each day. In his office note, the orthopedist wrote "there is slight discoloration of her right foot and she complains of burning pain but I do not think that she has RSD". I had no idea what RSD was or stood for at that time. I didn't see this note until two years later and he never mentioned it to me at all. I told the orthopedist that I couldn't tolerate the sneaker and he sent me to be measured for a MAFO (molded ankle foot orthodic). I now know that immobilizing the area with RSD makes the RSD worse. The MAFO did in fact made the burning worse. If you can't tolerate a sneaker how can you tolerate a sneaker with an appliance in it?

A year after the accident, Dr. E. decided that arthritis had developed in the joints surrounding the fractures. He told me that the only thing that would help would be cleaning out those joints and doing a bone fusion. Naively I believed him and had the procedure. This time around, it was four months in a cast followed by twelve weeks in the equalizer boot. Eight of those weeks were non-weight bearing on crutches again. I'd developed carpal tunnel syndrome from the stress on my wrists from the total of 16 weeks of crutch walking in 13 months. When I would tell Dr. E. about the burning pain being so severe, he would look at the latest x-ray and tell me that there was no physical reason for the pain. "The pain is in your head" as in his opinion there was no physical cause. I became very depressed. First of all I didn't know what was wrong with me. My family was getting annoyed with me, this fracture thing has been drawn out long enough. Friends faded away, again sick of hearing about that foot. They were sick of me canceling out on dates to get together because I was in too much pain. If I did get together with them then I was told that I wasn't "old self". Even friends who were nurses didn't know what to make of all of this. I began sinking lower and lower. " Hasn't that foot healed by now?" "Hasn't it been over a year now?" This is what they were saying; like I chose for this to happen?

I was seeing a therapist who was assigned to me by my health plan. She was a Licensed Social Worker. I told her that I was depressed. I told my family doctor that I was depressed. I was placed on an anti-depressant. This medication was prescribed by my primary physician. This too was a mistake; a psychiatrist should have been overseeing my psychiatric medication and care. However, my insurance company didn't cover anything other that a Licensed Social Worker unless they refer you to their psychologist who then refers you to their psychiatrist. The plan didn't want to cover psychiatric care so they made it really difficult to access.

It got to the point that I felt like I could not live like this any more. I tried to call the therapist. She was with patients and said that she would call me back. She didn't. I asked my oldest daughter to stay in my room and do her homework while I took my prescribed pain medication and went to sleep.

The next morning, the psychiatrist who worked with the Licensed Social Worked called and suggested that I needed a higher level of care. He suggested an inpatient psychiatric program at a local community hospital. Of course, this was the same local hospital where I used to work. (I also did my clinical rotation there in nursing school.) I agreed, not knowing what to do at this point. Was this pain real or was I crazy? I was assigned to a psychiatrist at the hospital who also worked at an affiliated local rehabilitation hospital. The first thing he did was to reassure me that the pain was real and not in my head. That was a huge relief. In over 18 months, he was the first one who actually acknowledged that this horrible burning pain that I was feeling was real and that I wasn't either making it up or that it was all in my head. I was discharged from the psychiatric unit in less than four days with hope for the first time in months. The psychiatrist, Dr A. recommended an outpatient chronic pain program at the rehabilitation hospital where he also worked. That was the turn in the right direction towards a diagnosis after nearly two years of no answers. During the chronic pain program, you see a physiatrist every other week. A physiatrist is a rehabilitation doctor. It was a multi-discipline approach to chronic pain.

I was evaluated by a psychologist, a physical therapist, and an occupational therapist. Part of the program was aqua therapy. I met one on one with a psychologist as well as attended group sessions where everyone in the group had chronic pain. They had bio-feedback sessions (biofeedback is the process of gaining greater awareness of many physiological functions primarily using instruments that provide information on the activity of those same systems, with a goal of being able to manipulate them at will. Some of the processes that can be controlled include brainwaves, muscle tone, skin conductance, heart rate and pain perception) which taught me how to manage my pain using my brain waves. The whole purpose of the program was to teach you to deal with your chronic pain without dependence on narcotics. I vividly remember several members of the group talking about previous narcotic dependency and how this program helped them manage their pain without narcotics. I was just beginning my journey with chronic pain but their words affected me greatly. Since weight bearing exercises were very difficult for me because of my foot; we concentrated on riding the reclining bicycle, core strengthening exercises, and just increasing my ability to stand for increased lengths of time. It was a very positive experience because I not only had a diagnosis but I knew that the pain was real and not in my head. I met others who had chronic pain and knew that I was not alone.

It was the physiatrist in the rehabilitation hospital who suggested that I might have RSD. As soon as I got home, I went on the Internet and plugged in RSD. Even as a nurse, I had never heard this term before! First I read all of the symptoms. They described me perfectly. They could have had me in front of them and been writing about me. Then I began reading articles. Many of the articles mentioned or were written by a specific doctor whose name seemed familiar to me. I called a friend who I'd known since 1983 and asked her if this doctor was her husband's boss. She said that he was. Although at that time, his boss was not taking on any new patients, my friend's husband got me an appointment with his director of pain management. It was this doctor who finally officially diagnosed me just over two years after my accident. For the purpose of this book we will call my friend Kathy, her husband Gilbert and the pain management doctor Dr. L.

Although this was just about the worst diagnosis that I could have received, I was so relieved to actually have a name for this and someone to tell me that it was not all in my head. I waited two months to see Dr L. In April of 1998, I saw Dr L who was dually board certified in neurology and anesthesiology. She confirmed my diagnosis of RSD and scheduled me for a Laser Doppler and Bier Block for the following month. By this time the burning had spread above the knee into the thigh and the Bier Block is not affective that high. We went ahead and did the Laser Doppler and Bier Block anyway but also scheduled a Lumbar Sympathetic Block. My friend Gil told me that one of the other PhD researcher's in his office found my Laser Doppler very unique and had a copy of it hanging in his office. The Laser Doppler shows the perfusion to the RSD affected limb and was one of the tools used in diagnosing RSD at that time. The Bier Block was meant to give pain relief. Since the burning had moved above the area that the block could cover, it only gave partial relief. Additionally, my situation was complicated by the fact that in addition to the burning pain from the RSD; I had the deep aching bone pain caused by the complex fractures and fusion. These RSD treatments were not designed to do anything for the bone pain.

In 1998, I had a series of blocks and a series of hospitalizations for pain management. The burning had spread from the right leg to my right arm, face, left arm, chest and left thigh. Fortunately it never spread to my left foot until recently. The pain was so intense that I could not tolerate the touch of clothing, a sheet or a breeze. I wore either a tank top and shorts (at home) or at work a sun dress and slippers.

Let's back track a little and talk about work. In 1996 during my accident, I had changed from patient care nursing to an administrative role, which still involved some home visits. It was a small home care company. I was on call 24 hours a day every other week. I was on back up to the person on call (just like the nurse who took over for me the night of my accident) when I wasn't the one on call. After the surgery to fuse my foot, I was smarter and went out on short term disability to take time to heal. It was a planned procedure so arrangements could be made to have someone cover for me unlike after the accident. Although it was very difficult dealing with this intense pain 24/7, working and raising two daughters (one of whom was blind), I could not even imagine not working. I loved being a nurse. Before my accident, I was in school to become a Nurse Midwife. I dropped out of the Nurse–Midwifery program realizing that after the injury, it was too much for me to go to school, work and take care of my family. I took a medical leave of absence from school hoping to go back to it.

In mid 1997, I made a job change. I had been offered the opportunity to get in on the ground floor of a new franchise home care agency opening in Philadelphia. I made the change. I still had not been diagnosed with RSD. Unfortunately for this employer and myself, my psychiatric hospitalization occurred during this employment and the opportunity to start the outpatient chronic pain program at Bryn Mawr Rehab; an eight week out patient program, occurred early on in this employment. I was let go because they felt that I could not fulfill my duties. I was crushed. I had never been fired from a job in my life. This was just another assault to my dignity that this injury had made.

After completing the Chronic Pain Program and while waiting the two months to see Dr L, I decided that with the knowledge that I had gained starting up this new franchise home care agency as well as the knowledge that I had gained in my previous home care positions, I would start my own home care agency. That gave me something to work towards and a renewed interest in life. It was not an easy road. Working with RSD isn't easy. There are doctor's appointments, treatments, the effects of medications or going without medications to have a clear head and the constant pain.

That brings us back to 1998. The business was underway, I was seeing Dr L and unforeseen by me, I would be spending a great deal of that year in the hospital. My receptionist would bring paperwork and payroll into me a the hospital. I had continuous epidurals, thoracic blocks, and IV Lidocaine, During one of these hospitalizations, after 24 hours of nurses and residents trying to get a peripheral IV in place, I was taken to the OR for what I had hoped would be a port. I argued with the surgeon telling him that I was a nurse and preferred a port to a Hickman, but he preferred a Hickman so it was a Hickman that I got. I It seemed that a treatment would work once and but not the second time. Finally the week of Thanksgiving, I was sent home after 10 days when no treatment worked.I was always feeling desperate to stop the pain. I was desperate to find a treatment that would work. I could't imagine living this way.

In six months when the Hickman needed to be replaced, I went to my own surgeon who had removed my appendix and gallbladder and she removed the Hickman and put in a port. I never wanted to be put through another 24 hours of IV sticks like I had during that hospitalization for the Lidocaine again!!

The next treatment that was presented to me was a medication pump. A trial was set up just after Christmas. We would try two different medications and if one worked, the surgery would be set for a permanent pump.

Bibuvicaine and Morphine were tried. Morphine had a better affect so in February 1999 a Medtronic pump was placed filled with Morphine. Over the next two years, combinations of mediations would be tried but over time the dosages would have to be increased and increased to get the same effect. Contrary to what I had been told, there was a systemic effect. The morphine made me sleepy, slowed my responses and did affect my work.

Ironically, on September 11, 2001, my professional world came to an end as I turned my home care business over to another pediatric company and stopped working. My RSD was affecting my gastrointestinal system. I was dealing with intermittent vomiting, and diarrhea. I had severe reflux. I could not sit at a desk top computer for any length of time without severe pain. I could not handle the on call schedule because I could not take anything for sleep as I would be impaired if I had to answer a medical question. The lack of sleep was making my pain worse.

The pump was no longer working. I had reached the maximum limits on the medications that my doctor was familiar with. Prior to that time, I only was these pumps used for children with Cerebral Palsy and filled with Baclofin to help with spasticity. Not as many people had them for pain management as they do today. There wasn't the experimentation with medications as there is today; at least not with the doctors that I was seeing. Dr L had moved on to another practice and my pump was being managed by the Dr who had been her fellow in 1998. He had joined her practice before she left.

While all of this was going on, I was also involved in a personal injury law suit against the auto insurance company of the driver who hit me 3/4/96. Even though she had been sited, she decided to change her story and denied that the accident was her fault. She didn't pay the ticket and there was a warrant out for her arrest. My insurance company paid out the current value of my car (which was only 10 months old so we lost out big on depreciation) and went after her insurance company for reimbursement. My husband hired a personal injury attorney because it had become obvious that this was going to be more than a simple fracture. So on top of trying to work, dealing with the pain and the medical issues, I had to deal with the legal issues. An insurance investigator was parked in front of my house. I lived on a cul de sac. My neighbor called the police to report a suspicious car parked in The neighborhood. She was told that it had permission to be there. The only thing that we could conclude was that it was there to spy on me.

There were depositions of myself, my husband, my doctors, and the other driver. I read Dr L's written statement. She listed my prognosis as poor. At the time, that puzzled me. I was sent to a doctor of the opposing insurance company's choice (an IME). I am not one to draw out my pain, but to stick straight to the facts. My attorney sent a nurse with me to document the appointment. This can be important because the independent medical exam is done by a doctor who works for the insurance company. Having a witness present validates your account of the exam. The physician had never come to the conclusion that anyone had RSD in the past. She gave me a thorough examination and submitted her report. She had really done her homework. She found an incident that had totally slipped my mind. Even if I had remembered it, I'm not sure that I would have made the link to my current problem. While working as a floor nurse five years earlier, I began having burning pain in my left foot. I saw a podiatrist who did a block, told me to stay off of my feet for a few days and the pain subsided. Much to everyone's surprise; she agreed that I had RSD. She felt that the incident five years ago was my first episode of RSD. It had gone into remission with the block. She felt that the reason it was so severe this time was because often after remission, when the RSD returns due to another injury, it comes back far worse. In my case, full body. Her only concern was the amount of edema that I had. Ironically, my own orthopedic was the only hold out. He never believed that I had RSD, but with their own independent physician agreeing with our expert that I had RSD, the insurance company could do nothing but to settle. That was a HUGE stress off of my mind. The law suit was a big stressor in my life. Trying to keep up with the lives of my daughters, husband and work all while in pain was overwhelming.

In October 2001, I received a call from my friend Gil. He said that Dr S was conducting a trial of a new treatment. This treatment was taking place in Germany and so far had very good results. He wanted to know if I was interested. I said that I was interested in learning more. Gil said that Dr. S's office would contact me for an appointment.

My father and his twin brother were born in Germany and spent their first 11 years there. I felt confident in the Germany health system. In many ways they were more progressive in Europe that here in the States. My appointment with Dr. S was postponed because he had been in Germany on 9/11 and was unable to fly back. Finally it was time for my appointment. I had met with Dr S many times. He had filled in for Dr L on many occasions when I had been hospitalized.

I learned that this treatment was to be a drug induced coma using a drug called Ketamine. The first two groups of two had been accompanied by Dr S, but after being trapped there this last trip, I would need to find my own physician to accompany me home. The other patient going at the same time was a physician and her father was a physician. He would accompany her home. I would have two weeks to make all of the arrangements. I would travel to Saarbrücken Germany. Dr. S explained that I would be placed in a Ketamine induced coma. My airway would be monitored as would my other vital signs. At this time, he hoped that this was a cure for RSD but it was too soon to tell. It was risky but as bad as my RSD was, it was my best chance. Dr S is a good salesperson but always adds in the risk factor, even if it's not in a tactful way. At the end of our conversation he said to me "some one is going to die from this". I left both excited and shaken. I knew that he wouldn't be sending patients if the dangers out weighted the potential benefits. Of course insurance wouldn't cover the costs which would be about $15K. I had my settlement from the law suit which

I could use for medical treatments. In addition to the treatment, there was the travel expense, hotel, meals, and the cost of taking a companion and flying a physician out to fly home with me. As a nurse, I knew what was involved in a medication induced coma. At that time, when I put Ketamine into the web browser the only thing that came up was special K and how it was used by attics.

Prior to the trip, I had to have some testing done. The first was a psychological and cognitive testing. Although we were weaning my morphine pump, they had to keep ringing the telephone in the room to wake me up as the testing was rather boring. Then they did some testing of temperature and sensation of the extremities that would be compared to tests done after the Ketamine. Ironically these same tests (except for the psychological/cognitive testing would be repeated when I got to Germany). The results of the testing and my response to the Ketamine were documented in a study co-authored by the doctors in Germany and Dr. S.

At the time my father was dying of ALS (Lou Gehrig's disease). He volunteered to go into a nursing home for two weeks so that my mom could go with me to Germany. That left my husband free to stay home and help my youngest daughter, Kim with her school work. My Uncle John (my father's twin) didn't feel comfortable with my mom being alone in Germany. He flew to Frankfort from San Francisco and a family friend who is an ER physician agreed to fly to Germany and return with us at the end of the treatment. Everything was all in place. At the last minute, I panicked. Those words that Dr S uttered "some one is going to die from this" were ringing in my head. I started screaming at a family dinner that I wasn't going. Here I was, a 46 year old woman, having a temper tantrum, saying that I wasn't going. I was screaming and crying. I was terrified that my girls wouldn't have a mother. I calmed down and once again started thinking rationally about it. Dr S wouldn't be sending his patients if he thought that it was that dangerous. As a nurse, I know the risks of a medically induced coma in an ICU. In this case, if my RSD were cured, the benefit would out weigh the risk. I got it out of my system and on October 26, 2001 my mother and I flew from Philadelphia International Airport to Frankfort.

We met up with my Uncle John in Frankfort where he had rented a car. It was a harrowing drive from Frankfort to Saarbruken. Saarbruken was a small town with a small shopping center. As my Uncle napped, my mother and I checked out the stores. I figured that I would be sleeping for a week any how. I was to have dinner with the two doctors who would be managing the treatment. This treatment was part of the studies that Dr S and the two German doctors were conducting. My mom and Uncle John had dinner together. I had dinner with Dr Roher, Dr Thomas, the other patient who was also named Nancy and her father Dr P. The dinner was a bit odd. Drs Roher and Thomas figured that we would want to meet the doctors whose care we were going to be under. They were right but since Nancy and I had never met either it just felt a bit strained. After dinner the doctors took us back to their lab and did the sensory tests themselves so that they would have a baseline before we started the treatment in the morning. I returning to the hotel.

It was a long sleepless night. As a nurse, I knew that during a medication induced coma, I would have an ART line (arterial line) to accurately measure my blood pressure and oxygen rate, a central line (I had hoped that they would use my port), a foley catheter to drain my urine, and cardiac monitoring. These were all things that I was familiar with although I had never had an arterial line before.

We reported to the hospital with our families and were taken to a room without the chance to say good bye. We discussed the fact that since I had severe reflux, they felt more comfortable intubating me. That actually made me more comfortable than just monitoring my breathing. They also told us that they found that by adding Versed and Clonidine they were hoping to eliminate the hallucinations that the first two groups experienced. That all sounded good to us. They were not familiar with my port so I accessed it. They put an IV in Nancy so she was asleep first.

Once my port was accessed, I too was off to sleep.

The only thing that I remember of the six days that I was in the coma was some unusual dreams. I had my daughters on my mind when I went to sleep, so the dreams were about them. They weren't scary and I knew that I was dreaming. I could tell myself that I was dreaming but I could not stop the dream. Then I remember my mother talking to me, but I could not talk to her. I felt too heavy to respond. I knew that she was there but could not respond. I guess that is when I was waking up. Evidently, I woke up 12 hours after the other Nancy. My wrists were tied down so that I wouldn't pull anything out as I was waking up. I wasn't afraid. Once I was fully awake, things progressed fairly quickly. I began sitting up, took a short walk, showered, etc. I had NO pain; NO pain at all. They reset my pump again and wrote down that it needed to be refilled and decreased December 7th. Nancy and I were moved to a regular room for one day and given PT. We were given the sensory testing again all for the sake of the research study.

Dr David (our family friend) came in to visit and speak with Dr Rohr and Dr Thomas about the treatment and what to watch for on the trip home. I've known Dave since we were kids. He's a great guy. He was very interested in how the Ketamine worked. The next morning I was released. We hired a car to take us to Frankfort. We used a wheel chair as I was still very week from the week of bed rest and the coma. The airport in Frankfort post 9/11 was very different than those in the US. There were armed guards with riffles. We boarded our flight and arrived home on Veterans Day 2001.

Unfortunately there was some sort of mixup with the pump. Thanksgiving weekend, it started beeping, which means that either the battery is dying or the pump is empty. I could't get a hold of the doctor who was managing the pump over the holiday weekend. It beeped all weekend. That Monday morning, I called the doctor and he set up an appointment for Tuesday. At the appointment, he said that the pump was in fact empty and that the doctors in

Germany must have miscalculated the refill date. He refilled it at a lower dosage as per Dr S previous orders rather than calling him to see what he wanted to do since the pump had been empty over a long weekend.

After the appointment, I stopped by my parents' house to take my dad his favorite meal; a pizza and Breyer's Chocolate Ice Cream. That cheered my dad up. I began feeling nauseated. I stayed for a while and then said that I would be back the next day to help out my mom as I had been doing. During that night, I became intensely ill vomiting intractably. I sent my husband over to help my mother in my place. I thought that it was a stomach bug. While taking a nap that afternoon, my father stopped breathing and passed away. I wasn't able to be there. I was still vomiting intractably. Now I was getting dehydrated and needed to go to the ER. Jim stayed with my mom until arrangements had been made. That should have been me. I was feeling horrible that I wasn't there with my dad to say goodbye. When Jim got home, he then had to take me to the ER. They pumped me full of fluids and anti emetics (anti-nausea drugs) and sent me home on no medications. As soon as we got home, I vomited in the sink. I vomited for a second night. In the morning back to the ER we went. None of us related it to the pump refill. I went to a local hospital, not the hospital where the doctor was who refilled the pump practices in Philadelphia. I was admitted to the local hospital I was given IV fluid and anti emetics for several days until they could get me drinking clear fluids and progress to full liquids and eventually solids. When I saw Dr. S, he said that it was morphine over dose and that the doctor who managed my pump should never have refilled it once it ran out. Of course the doctor who refilled it said that it was morphine withdrawal. I guess we'll never know. The worst part was that I wasn't with my parents when my father passed. I didn't get to say good by to my dad. Dr S was surprised that all of this didn't undo the Ketamine coma treatment because needle sticks for IVs and blood work (the German doctors had broken my port) and the stress of my father's death could trigger a relapse. My father died just two weeks after my return from Germany.

It was December 26th, 2001 when the burning in my foot returned. Dr S had taken me off of all of my RSD medications. I called him immediately and he resumed my medications. Slowly the burning pain returned. At this time, there were no "booster" Ketamine programs in the US. The other Nancy had been a surgical resident at Copper Hospital and Trauma Center in Camden NJ. Her pain was returning as well. She got the head of anesthesiology at Cooper Hospital to do outpatient Ketamine under Dr S's guidance for the two of us. Thus, in February 2002, the first outpatient Ketamine treatment program was born in the busy pre-op section of a major trauma OR. It consisted of the two of us who were overseen by the anesthesia department of Cooper under the direction of Dr S. We were not permitted to eat or drink after midnight. We were given 12 Ketamine infusions in February and March. The burning went from a 7 back to a 0, only to return again. It was still a learning process. During these outpatient infusions, an IV was started (until I got a new port) we were given pre-medications of glycol (to dry up your saliva), Versed (to prevent hallucinations) and Zophran (to prevent nausea). The IV was up and ran over a period of four hours but the entire process usually took about six hours from signing the consent, meeting with the anesthesiologist to filling out the pain form at the end. You had to have someone drive you to and from. Since it was over an hour's drive from my house in Downingtown PA to Cooper in Camden NJ; my ride would have to wait there for that six hours and read in the waiting room. Camden isn't exactly an area where you'd want to go out and take a stroll. Fortunately, my retired Uncle had volunteered to be my driver. He lived about twenty minutes from our house. He had to pick me up at 6:30 in order for us to get there in time. I of course paid for the gas and tolls. I was so grateful that my Uncle was able to do this for me as my husband travels for a living.

I had renewed hope following the coma and subsequent Ketamine infusions. I retook my GREs (as five years had gone by since I originally took them) and started back to school to become a nurse midwife. I did great with the book work. When it came time for clinical, I came to the realization that there was no way that my foot was going to tolerate being on my feet for clinical. Crushed, I withdrew from school once again.

In August, we tried an inpatient admission to Hahnemann for Ketamine based on compassionate plea. I was in Hahnemann August 6 – 16. The Ketamine was titrated to 30 mg/hr. I was awake as anesthetic doses of Ketamine are not permitted in the US. The hospital admission was followed by outpatient Ketamine at Cooper on August 22, 29 and 30 as well as September 30, October 1, 2, 3, and 4th. I had an additional treatment November 5, 6, 7 and 8th. These out patient infusions didn't seem to be able to keep my burning pain at bay because after the holidays, I ended up right back in the hospital for another inpatient Ketamine infusion. During this time, other people were going to Germany and having a variety of outcomes. You can see the full study in appendix D Efficacy of Ketamine in Anesthetic Dosage for the Treatment of Refractory Complex Regional Pain Syndrome: An Open–Label Phase II Study.

Over 2002, the Morphine in the pump was completely weaned and replaced with saline until the battery failed and stopped. I chose not to have it removed as I didn't want to have another surgery at this time. It wasn't causing any problems just sitting there; so just sit that is what it did. It was no longer influencing my medical care or my pain management.

January 3 – 13, 2003, I was admitted to Hahnemann for a Ketamine infusion that was titrated to 40 mg/hr, During these admissions, there was no contact by phone with your family or friends. My husband travels for a living. He was only able to call into the nurses' station and get a report on my condition. Both of my daughters were off to college, but were still home on there semester break. They could come in and visit for short periods of time but mostly they wanted to hang out with their friends. They had spent Christmas with me and I didn't want to hamper their winter break.

It was very difficult for me to get a ride to Cooper from Downingtown (over an hour's drive) to have that person wait the six hours that it took for them to get the monitors hooked up, the IV started, the premeds given and the infusion started, then drive me home. My Uncle had been doing it; but he had had an accident and fell down his steps breaking his neck. Fortunately he wasn't totally paralyzed but it was a long recovery and he was no long capable of making the long drive. Jim traveled. My mom didn't drive and my cousins all worked. I decided that I needed to take a break from Ketamine for a while due to the transportation issues.

At this point, I was seeing a psychiatrist who specialized in chronic pain. She was a board certified Pain Management Doctor as well as a Board Certified Psychiatrist. She had been referred by Dr S. I found her easy to talk to. We went back to the beginning of when I'd been injured and worked our way to the present over a long period of time. She helped me deal with the repeating issues with family and friends and the fact that they really didn't get what it was like to have RSD; expecting more from me than I was physically capable of giving. We worked on other issues that are not relevant to my RSD. I ended up seeing her for a total of 7 years. I learned a lot about myself from her and through our therapy. I highly suggest that everyone with chronic pain find a therapist who specializes in treating patients with chronic pain because our situation is different than the average psychological patient. It was an important part of my learning to live with my RSD.

By January 2004, the follow up Ketamine outpatient treatments were in place and protocols were established. They were no longer being done in the pre-op but rather in what used to be a suite at Cooper. Except for the fact that my allodynia was gone, my RSD pain was as bad as ever. A joint decision between Dr S, my psychiatrist, and the German doctors was made that I should go back to Germany for a second coma treatment. This time my husband would come with me as both of my daughters were in college. Dr S's study was still going on but I had the physical studies done in Germany. This time, I knew the doctors and I knew what to expect. I wasn't going to let them use my port so I let them put in a central line like they do with the other patients. I asked my husband to keep a journal but I won't bother to share it with you because it is all about what was going on in the world, not about the medical things going on.. I don't know why I expected any thing else as he is not a medical person. The big difference this time is that we were given nasogastric feedings; which we were not given last time. Everyone was intubated now. My roommate this time was a 21 year old college student. Jim was able to have dinner with his mother and share cabs to visit us. Physicians were no longer required to accompany patients home either.

January 19, 2004 we arrived at the hospital at 9 am for the pre-Ketamine testing. This testing involves testing your tolerance to heat and cold as well as measuring the temperature of your extremities. After the testing was complete, we were taken into a small room where a peripheral IV was started to put us to sleep and our families were sent home. From there, we were transferred to the ICU where: a central line was put in, an arterial line was put in, a foley catheter was placed, and cardiac leads were placed. As we were more heavily sedated; we were intubated. At that point, the Ketamine infusion could begin along with drugs to protect your brain from hallucinations. In my case I was getting Midazolam, Clonidin and Fentynl. I was getting 4 mg per kg of my weight per hr of Ketamine.

January 24, 2004 they began tapering off the medications in an effort to wake us up. My roommate was awaking more quickly than I was. January 25, my husband said that if he called my name, I would open my eyes but other wise, I was still pretty much out of it. I was trying to pull out the tubes, so my hands were restrained. About 4 pm that afternoon I fully woke up and they were able to remove the breathing tube and put me on oxygen. I could answer simple questions but was very sleepy. Monday January 26th, 2004, when my husband came in I was sitting in a chair and I, as he put it, "went into my discharge mode". The feeding tube was out. I had had my husband bring me bottled water as I had learned from my first trip to Germany that they drank carbonated water. I preferred what they called flat water; which had to be purchased at the store. I was very thirsty and started on clear liquids such as broth and jello. I had no recollection of seeing Jim on Sunday at all. The doctors said that they hoped to move me out of ICU the next day. My husband left me with my headphones on, my chapstick and my German-English/English-German Dictionary at my bedside. They allowed him to stay later than the 6 p.m. visiting hours. Tuesday January 27th, I was moved to a regular room where I had an elderly German woman as a roommate who spoke very little English. My diet was advanced and I was able to get out of bed more easily. From now on it was just a matter of advancing my diet and rebuilding my strength to prepare for the trip home. Wednesday January 28th, I showered, had my central line pulled and continued to walk around the unit as I regained my strength. After some tests on my foot Thursday and Friday to see if there was anything that could be done to help with the bone pain, it was decided that nothing could be done but to reduce the bone pain with opiates, keep the foot quite so that it wouldn't aggravate the RSD. I was discharged Friday and we started our journey back home on Saturday.

It was back to the outpatient treatments at Cooper on a regular basis to maintain the effects of the coma Ketamine. In February, I went twice a week for four weeks. We hired a car service to take me to and from and my mother in law who lived with us was home with me at night. I still had no family member to do the driving. It was becoming quite expensive to have the car service drive me to Camden when my husband was out of town. When he was in town, he would drop me off and I would wait in the lobby until he was finished work at the end of the day. It seemed that when I was getting Ketamine, my entire life revolved around the Ketamine. It took the remainder of that week for me to recover from the two days of infusions so essentially for those four weeks, my life was Ketamine. The Ketamine wasn't holding. So in March 2004, I went back inpatient at

Hahnemann for a 6 day inpatient admission. This would be the last Ketamine that I would get for a while.

My alodenia was 100% better, except occasionally on my foot. I think that I was expecting too much. When I would come home from Germany, I would be pain free or close to pain free but that wouldn't hold. My foot would start back up almost immediately. Nothing would keep that from happening or could control that. I came to the realization that this was the best that I could get. If the pain were confined to my foot with a little in my face (for some reason my foot and face had become connected) then that was the best that I could be. I needed to stop chasing after something better because at this point in time there wasn't anything better. I needed to stop being a "professional" patient and get back to living my life.

I found things to do to distract myself from the pain. I utilized the relaxation exercises that I had used in childbirth and learned to pace myself. In August 2005, I sent my records to doctor in Palm Bay FL who had been recommended by my roommate on the second trip to Germany. They managed RSD pain with trigger point injections. He felt that they could help me. For five days every three months, I would travel to FL with my husband for the injections. They really made a difference.

In February 2006, Dr H (my FL doctor) suggested that we move to FL. He felt that every time that I came, he was only able to get me to a certain point. Once I went back to the colder climate, the good that he did would slowly be undone. Since my husband only needs a computer, phone, fax and airport to do his job, we moved to Orlando FL in June 2006. I continued to see Dr H until he moved his practice out of the area in 2009. I found myself looking for a pain management doctor in Orlando. Before moving his practice, Dr H suggested an inpatient Ketamine treatment with Dr S. I got great results after the 6 day infusion.

In 2008 I was diagnosed with a ruptured lumbar disc and uterine cancer. I had the total hysterectomy first followed a month later by a fusion of my back. It was a very rough year. A complication of the hysterectomy and lymph node removal, my bladder stopped working effectively. I was not able to completely empty my bladder and had to start using a catheter to empty my bladder.

In late 2009, Dr C was recommended to me by my primary doctor. After reviewing my records, his suggestion was to implant a spinal column stimulator. I should have contacted Dr S and asked his opinion but I didn't. I had the trial of the stimulator. For this, they place the leads on your back, tape them down and you wear the device around your waist like a fanny pack. I got good results from the trial so a date was set for surgery.

You are awake for the first part of the surgery. They stimulate different areas of your spinal nerves until they find the one that sends the tingling pulsation to the area that it is needed. Once they locate the placement, they put you to sleep to implant the battery pack and tunnel the wires. For eight weeks after the surgery you can not bend, twist or turn to prevent the leads from migrating.

I asked Dr C if it would be ok to go on vacation a month after the surgery. We had the trip scheduled before the surgery was scheduled. He didn't see it as a problem. We went to CA. One morning, I woke up and the bed was saturated. I had not peed the bed, so where did it come from. I asked my husband to look at my back and the incision where that they made to put the stimulator in was red and the discharge was coming from there. I called Dr C. He said that I needed to go to the ER. He gave me his cell phone number and we preceded to the hospital that the hotel recommended. I saw a physician's assistant when I arrived. I told him that my surgeon wanted to speak to him. They waited until 11:00 Eastern time to call Dr C. He told him that it was just suture irritation. Fortunately Dr C knew that I was a nurse and what I described to him could not have been from suture irritation. Dr C asked the physician's assistant in CA to put me on oral antibiotics. Fortunately we were going home in 48 hours.

As soon as we were home, I went to Dr C's office when it opened. The nurse practitioner called Dr C who was doing procedures out of the office. He told her to find me a hospital bed and to consult with an infectious disease doctor. Within the hour, I was admitted to the hospital. IV antibiotics were started and the wound cultured. The infectious disease doctors wanted the device removed by Dr C wanted to see if the antibiotics would be effective. The wound started to open up and you could see the wires. The devise was taken out and I was sent home on IV antibiotics for a total of 8 weeks. The wound could not be sutured because of the infection so I had wound care for weeks provided by a home care nurse.

In the fall of 2011, I took a nasty fall. Before hand my RSD had been contained to my right foot and occasionally my face as a result of the Ketamine infusions. I contacted Dr S and he arranged for me to be admitted in January 2012 for inpatient Ketamine. Following the inpatient admission, he recommended a doctor in Miami to do the follow up boosters. The Miami anesthesiologist feels that it is the dose that is important and not the length of the infusions. He gave me an infusion that was 2 mg of Ketamine per kilogram of weight for four hours five days in a row. I got excellent relief from this treatment.

Back in 1996 and 1997, I developed carpal tunnel syndrome from crutch walking. It remained tolerable over the years. To compensate for my right foot, I often used my upper body more than the average person. By September of 2011 my right hand would go numb after minimal use. Dr C did an EMG. An EMG is a test where they put two needles into your extremity at different points and add an electrical impulse between the two to measure how well the nerve carries the impulse. The test revealed that my carpal tunnel syndrome had progressed to severe in my right hand (I'm right handed) and moderate in my left.

While I was in Philadelphia for my inpatient Ketamine in January 2012, I discussed these results with Dr S. Without surgery, the carpal tunnel syndrome will cause me to lose further use of my hand. With the surgery, there is a 50% spread rate from the surgery. Dr S felt that by having Ketamine during the surgery and immediately thereafter, my odds would be greatly improved. June 20, 2012 I had the carpal tunnel release under Ketamine. It was supposed to be followed by 5 outpatient infusions. When I got to Miami, I was informed that they were running out of Ketamine. So instead of 5 days of 6 hour infusions, I got 3 four hour infusions. It was not enough to stay off spread to my right wrist/hand. I began a series of out patient infusions which has calmed my hand down but it still swells and burns on bad weather days.

Sure, if I had to do things over again, I may have made some different treatment choices. I didn't know that ice would cause me more problems and used to use it regularly when I was burning. Would not I have had the spinal cord stimulator up in. After my foot fusion surgery, I got multiple opinions from other foot and ankle orthopedist and none of them brought up RSD. If I'd been diagnosed sooner....well I wasn't and this is the way things are! After over 16 years with RSD, I still miss nursing but I have found a way to utilize my nursing skills by helping others with RSD. I am the administrator of an on line support group. My life is good as I will not let RSD rule my life. I have finally learned how to pace myself. There are special occasions where I over do things knowing that I will pay for it later. Some things are worth the pain afterwards. I've been married for 34 years to a man who looks at my RSD this way; neither of us envisioned me having RSD. These are the cards that we were dealt and we need to make the best of the blessings that we do have. Our youngest daughter and son in law are expecting our first grandchild. I am no longer obsessed with finding a treatment that will take it all away. If my foot and face are the only places that I am burning, then it's a great day! When RSD rears it's ugly head full body, I make the necessary arrangements for Ketamine if it lasts longer than two weeks. I use a wheel chair for anything that involves a lot of walking. It enables me to travel with my husband and do things that I would not otherwise be able to do if I were walking. I got over feeling strange about being in a wheel chair along time ago. I have more good days than bad ones. I remain optimistic that researchers will some day figure this disease out but I am not going to stop living my life waiting for it to happen!

Emily's Story

I am 33 years old and I have had RSD for over year now. I had a punch biopsy in my left breast to rule out skin cancer, it was very soon after that I knew something was very wrong. (negative for skin cancer it was contact dermatitis) The type of pain in my Left Breast was like no other I have ever felt or experienced. Soon I started to get the "burn" and the "bees" stinging me. The pain then traveled to my hands/ wrist area (more so the right than left and my fingers would lock up) and my right knee (deep bone ache).
My pain management put me on a combo of non-narcotics and narcotics to help with the pain. He then recommended epidurals for the constant breast pain. I had 2 of them with no benefits. At that point he did not have many suggestions other than increasing my narcotic medications or a Spinal Cord Stimulator (SCS). As a Registered Nurse I knew there had to be other options. I soon realized that I was going to have to be my own advocate. It was difficult and I had a steep learning curve but I did not give up. I knew very quickly that I was not going to be able to handle this type of pain for the rest of my life. I started researching and talking with anyone that knew anything about RSD and treatments. I read about Ketamine, SCS or other types of Blocks. It was during this time I discovered Calmare Therapy.
First, I would like to explain to you what Calmare is. Calmare therapy is non-invasive, painless, and drug free. It is used to treat various types of chronic pain, including RSD/CRPS, Intractable Cancer Pain, Failed Back Surgery Syndrome, Sciatic and Lumbar Pain, Post-Herpetic Neuralgia, Brachial Plexus Pain, and Peripheral Neuropathies.

It is a biophysical methodology rather than biochemical (no drugs). The Calmare machine, MC-5A, scrambles that message that the D nerves fibers are sending to your brain saying "PAIN, PAIN, PAIN" to "NO PAIN, NO PAIN, NO PAIN". The electrical impulses communicate with the D nerve pain fibers that have the memory. It is recommended you go through 10 sessions because you need that repetition that allows your brain to be "re-trained". When I speak of the 10 sessions, each session lasts of anywhere from 35-60 minutes a day. (This depends on the physician; my doctor did 60 minute sessions). Most people schedule their 10 sessions of Calmare therapy, usually starring on Monday and going through Friday (5) and then have off Saturday and Sunday and then finish the next week (5).

During your first session you will meet with your Calmare Therapy Physician. They will do their first consultation and map out your pain areas. Once this is done, your physician will place sticky electrodes near your pain areas on the same Dermatomes. A dermatome is an area of skin supplied by sensory neurons that arise from a spinal nerve ganglion. Your physician will determine how many electrodes will be place in that area. For example, for my first treatment, I had 4 electrodes around my breast, and then each electrode is connected to a lead that is connected to the MC-5A Calmare Machine. Your physician will start off with the very lowest setting a move up very slowly. It does take a little time for the body to acclimate to the electric impulse. It was not painful to me; actually it was relaxing and made me want to sleep. Before each session you will rate your pain in each area and then after the treatment you will do the same. With my experience, my pain rating always decreased from the beginning to the end.

It is a good idea to bring something to read or music to listen to. My dad came with me and we had a great time catching up. (He also went through Calmare therapy for his Back pain, sciatic pain, and numb foot)

As far as your medications are concerned, it is advised that you are off drugs like Gabapentin, Cymbalta, and Lyrica. Please consult your doctor when getting off these types of drugs. All of your other drugs are safe and when you starting getting relief the doctor will work with you to titrate off some of your stronger pain medications/narcotics. You can NOT receive Calmare therapy if you have a Pacemaker or SCS that is turned in the On mode.

A little background on the Calmare Therapy, there are only a few doctors who do this therapy because it is new to the US. It has only been here and FDA approved for 2 years. It was invented in Italy and has been used there for many years. It was developed by Professor Giuseppe Marineo in Rome, Italy. He researched chronic pain for over 24 years. At this time, insurance is not covering Calmare Therapy; however, there is a big study being done at a few clinics. I know at Mayo Clinic they are using Calmare therapy on cancer patients and their pain. So there is an insurance code but it is only for cancer patients and not for chronic pain patients. Cross our fingers that all insurances will pick this up to treat chronic pain, specifically RSD/CRPS. It is so much cheaper in the long run when you think how much money you spend on all your mediations monthly. Calmare Therapy rates depend on the physician. With that being said I, have seen rates ranging from $1,000-$3,000 for the full 10 sessions and consultation. This will need to be discussed with your physician.

The physician who treated me was Dr. Greg Sheehan, located in Glastonbury, CT. His website is www.ctprc.com. Dr. Sheehan was excellent and I highly recommend him. But with that being said, I have talked with people who have had calmare with other doctors and they all sound great too. Dr. Cooney is located in NJ and Dr. D'Amato is located in RI.

For more information on Calmare Therapy please go to find a list of doctors and where they practice, www.calmarett.com.

I have gone through Calmare Therapy twice both times with Dr. Sheehand. I had my first Calmare Therapy treatment in Oct. 2011. My pain levels were 8-9 out of a 10. We concentrated on my left breast, right hand and right knee. I felt relief within the first few sessions. The RSD burn was the symptom that I noticed decreased the most. Also my fingers were locking up less. This was such a huge deal and I was so relieved that this was working. My pain levels when I left was at 0, 1–2 (at tops) out of a 10.

I went through 9 treatments/sessions (1 treatment was canceled due to a snow storm). When I arrived via plane from Arizona to Connecticut I was in a wheelchair, due to my pain. I also used a cane to help with ambulation. When I left for Arizona I walked onto the plane all on my own (without my cane). My pain levels stayed low and it felt so good to be out of that horrible pain I was in 24/7.

I also want to mention that my dad accompanied me to Connecticut and he also went through Calmare Therapy for his Back pain, sciatic pain, and numb foot. It was so neat having my dad not only be there with me but also going through the same therapy at the same times as me. He also had great results and was pretty much pain free when we flew home. Currently he is now having back pain again but he has not had any booster treatments and has been living a very active lifestyle.   He is currently looking into trying the Spinal Cord Stimulator Trial.

The biggest side–effect that I personally experience after Calmare Therapy was fatigue and this is normal too. Again go slow.

Unfortunately, my RSD spread to my left knee in Decemeber 2011. I was also having some pain in my original areas. I had to fly back to Connecticut this time with my mom in Feb. 2012. Again, I arrive in a wheelchair due to my pain. When I walked I had to use a cane. I was having the same type of "burn/bees" and deep bone ache that was constant. Before my Calmare I rated my pain 8 out of 10 (with the pain getting up to a 10 at times). I went through 10 treatments/sessions and when I left my pain was less than 2 out of 10. In addition to treating my new left knee pain we did boosters to the right knee and both the hands/wrist area. We did not treat my original Left breast area, however I wished we had after the fact.

It is advised and very important to take it very easy after treatment. You need to give your body time as it has been "re-trained".

Yes I would recommend trying Calmare therapy as it is non-invasive treatment and it does help but you have to have money to pay for this treatment upfront, as I stated above insurance is still not covering this treatment. In my opinion I think that most people with RSD with have to get Boosters at some point.
It is unfortunate that there is no cure for RSD however; Calmare Therapy does decrease the pain significantly. Some people will need to get boosters treatments or have a new area treated.

In May my RSD pain was back. We did not have the money to go back to get another booster. I transferred to a different Pain Management doctor to see if he had any different ideas. We tried different medications some really didn't have any benefits, such as Lyrica. We just recently started Lumbar Sympathetic Blocks to treat my Left knee pain. I have gone through 2. The first one did decrease my pain for a few days (both the burn and deep bone ache). So far I have not gotten any relief from my second block, however it was just given less than 2 days ago.

Overall I am not doing well. I am in the process of filing for Social Security Disability and have had to hire a SSD lawyer, as I have been unable to work for over a year now. I was working for a hospice company as their Admission's RN. I loved my job and would do anything to get back to work. I was healthy before I got RSD .
Many of my RSD/CRPS symptoms have gotten worse over the year and I have been very ill. My illness has caused my RSD/CRPS to flare. I have also been diagnosed with new conditions since I was diagnosed RSD/CRPS. I will explain: (from Emily's Journal)

My RSD/CRPS that started in my Left Breast, then traveled to my hands/wrist area (more so the right than left and my fingers would lock up) and my right knee (deep bone ache), has now spread into my Left knee. I have extreme pain in my Left knee. When I use the word extreme, its due to the intense "deep bone ache" and "burn" I feel (it feels like your arm is in a fire and you can't take it out). I also get "the bees" from time to time, especially on the Left Breast (when I use the description of the bees, it feels like 100 bees sting you in a certain area and then turn around and stab you). The pain is so intense that it paralyzes me, for example if I am doing something or having a conversation , I freeze and close my eyes and just try to breathe slowly and wait for it to pass. I take Morphine 3 times a day (Pain), Hydromorphone (Diluadid) as needed for breakthrough (Pain), Naproxen twice a day (anti–inflammatory), Nortriptyline twice a day (Nerve Pain, depression, anxiety), and Lidocaine 5% Gel as need to put on my knee or breast

1. I get Allodynia, where any normal touch or sensation causes pain. This is occurs in all my RSD areas, especially my Left knee. I also experience Hyperalgesia, Hyperesthesia, and Lancinating pain. All of these symptoms seem to have increased and gotten worse since Jan./Feb.

2. My left knee will swell at night and now I am having skin changes, mottling.

3. I also had pain in my hands/wrists when last reported and my fingers would lock up/spasms and swell, however this seems to have gotten worse. It takes longer in the morning to get my fingers moving and unlocked then it did a few months ago. I always wear my compression gloves, since they seem to help prevent the locking of the joints.

4. In addition to that intense pain, I have muscle and joint ache and stiffness. My joints and muscles will ache so badly and it is impossible to get comfortable. It feels like I have the flu every day.

5. I use a cane daily to do all of my activities due to my pain and weakness/fatigue/exhaustion.

6. My weakness/fatigue/exhaustion is pretty extreme. I

know that I stated this in my last report but it too has gotten worse. I have zero energy and endurance. I am on the sofa or in my bed most of each day. I have terrible fatigue and exhaustion

7. I'm having increased anxiety and now I am feeling depression related to my RSD/CRPS and the situation I am in. I am also experiencing panic attacks. I can't stop crying and having emotional break downs multiple times a week. I am more irritable and get irritated easily, getting into more arguments with my family. My Pain Managment doctor started me on a new medication, Nortriptlyine. It is supposed to help with pain, anxiety and depression. I know I would benefit from working with someone and having someone to talk too. I had been working with Pain Psychologist (but it has been many months since I have seen her). RSD/CRPS is a struggle every day. I am scheduled to see a psychiatrist this week.

8. My insomnia has gotten worse and take medications to help sleep at night, Ambiene and Melatonin.

9. My RSD/CRPS is causing extreme temperature changes. I had experienced this some in the earlier months but it has also gotten worse. I am either freezing/shivering or I am very hot and sweating. I now dress in layers so that I can add or take off to try and get comfortable. For example, showers are miserable because they alter my body temperature; it sometimes takes up to 30 minutes after I get out of the shower for my body to adjust. My body will be so freezing cold/goose bumps but yet I am dripping sweat from my forehead and back area

10. My low immune system. I get recurrent infections especially throat infections. I see an Infectious Disease physician. I take many supplements daily.

11. I have developed Hypothyroidism. They also found 2 cysts on my Thyroid Gland. I am now being prescribed medication for this. I take Synthroid daily.

My CRPS has been elevated for a few months now, indicating the amount of inflammation I have in my body. It is now up to 22 indicating high inflammation body wide.

My menstrual cycle has decreased. Before RSD/CRPS I had 28 day cycles that lasted 5 days long. In the last 3 months, it usually last 1 day at the most or I don't get it at all.

I still continue to have pain in my Left Breast with the "bees" stinging me and pain in my right knee that comes and goes (This has not changed)

Hypertension and Tachycardia. I am now seeing a Cardiologist, my medications were increased. I have had multiple EKG's, holter monitor test and Echo. The test show that my HR/BP being elevated is related to my RSD/CRPS due to it affecting the sympathetic nervous system, pain, and being so de-conditioned. I take Atenolol daily.

Severe Constipation. I take Mirlax daily. I also take Milk of Magnesium or laxatives as need.

Here is a list of my physical and mental limitations since I was diagnosed with RSD/CRPS:

* I cannot lift more than 5 lbs (do not have the strength)

*I cannot squat because it hurts my kenes.

*I cannot bend because it hurts my back.

* I cannot stand more than 5 minutes (pain/fatigue/weakness/endurance). I also have a shower chair in my bath tub so that I can sit down

* I cannot reach because straightening out my arms, causes the muscles and joints to ache.

* I cannot walk more than 5 minutes (pain/fatigue/weakness/endurance). I now use a Cane to Ambulate. If I walk any more than 5 minutes, I have to sit down for 5-10

minutes and rest. I have also noticed that my feet will swell and change color if I am standing on them for any length of time. If I will be doing anything long distance I have to rent a wheelchair.

* Stair Climbing is very difficult for me. I can barely do 1 flight of stairs, it can take me 5 minutes or longer. I have to take multiple breaks before I can reach the top (pain/fatigue/endurance/weakness).

* My short-term memory is more pronounced and I have a hard time concentrating daily (pain medications/poor concentration/foggy mind). This used to be only on my bad days.

*I having an increasingly difficult time completing task on a daily basis (due to pain/fatigue/ weakness/endurance/poor concentration).

*I am having an increasingly difficult time concentrating on a daily basis (pain medications/foggy mind).

*I am having an increasingly difficult time using my hands especially in the morning when my fingers and joints in the hands are locked up. I also get pain in my hands and wrist at times, this cause difficultly in typing and writing.

*I am having an increasingly difficult time understanding. I never had a problem with this before my RSD/CRPS. Sometimes things have to be explained twice or in a different way for me to understand. (Poor Concentration/Poor Memory/Foggy mind/pain medications)

*I can sit for 20-25 minutes with my feet hanging down, but after that point I start getting pain. I have to elevated my legs, specifically the Left Leg or my pain will increase significantly.

I am having an increasingly time following instructions, if they are not written down, I have an extremely hard time doing this (Poor Concentration/Poor Memory/Foggy mind/

pain medications).

I am having an increasingly difficult time getting along with others because of my increased depression and anxiety. It makes it hard for me to deal with people at times, even my family. I get irritable and irritated very easily. I have also had panic attacks. I am having emotional break downs a few times a week, where I can't stop crying. RSD and all the changes have affected all aspects of my life and become huge stressors.

As stated above, before RSD/CRPS, I was able to care for myself 100 percent, I lived alone, I worked full time, I was able to drive I cared for my 2 cats, I belonged to a gym, I went out on the weekends and did fun activities. I had a very full life. RSD/CRPS has changed all aspects of my life. I have tired many different medications, epidurals, Calmare therapy, and Sympathetic Blocks and nothing has profoundly helped me. It is very easy to get wrapped up in this disease as it affects all aspects of your body/mind/spirit, but you have to fight each day so that doesn't happen. It is also a goal to try to learn something new about RSD/CRPS each week so that I will always be up to date with the new treatments, medications, etc etc.

Kathryn
Columbus, OH

Hello. My name is Katie. I am 32 yrs old. I am a registered nurse and certified as a CGRN. I work in gastroenterology, which has been my passion for the past 10 yrs. It is weird that something I love, is also the one thing that has changed my life forever. To explain this, we have to go back a few years to May 30, 2008. I remember the day clearly. I was working for a co-worker, so he could take his family on a camping trip for the weekend. This was not my normal day to work.... It was a day I traded, to help a co-worker. Early in the morning on this day, we were transporting a patient back from a procedure done in radiology on the second floor of the hospital. We were going around a turn bringing the patient and equipment back to our unit. As we rounded the turn, the co-worker in front of me stopped suddenly. This caused a chain reaction of events. The cart that a person was pushing behind me sandwiched me between the patient on a gurney and the equipment cart that was being pushed behind me. The equipment cart behind me caught the bottom of my left heel...turned my foot completely upside down, and the cart remained on top of my foot for approximately 30 seconds. I knew immediately that I injured my foot....to the severity, I never would know at that time. But, this day forever changed my life. I had a lot of anger, as I was not supposed to be there that day. But, I put patients and others first. I was helping a co-worker out so he could go camping with his family. And, this is the day that my life was changed forever.

I was taken to employee health/occupational medicine. My left foot was screaming, I was in so much pain. I started to swell immediately. I was wheeled over for x-rays. Before I even made it back to the employee health doctor, she met me at the door and said I had fractured my foot pretty badly. I had 4 fractures: anterior calcaneal, cuboid, 2 navicular fractures(all avulsion fractures, meaning the bone was twisted and turned and pulled off to break it). I asked about the possible ligament damage, with my background I am fully aware what can and can't be seem with just an x-ray. That we wouldn't know for a few more weeks. The doctor made a request for me to see orthopedic surgeon, of which I couldn't get into for 6 weeks post- injury. I was a workers compensation patient....what could I do????....nothing. She placed me in a big boot, placed me on crutches, and told me to stay off of it until I could be seen by the orthopedic surgeon.

In the weeks that followed, I started to notice that my foot was extremely sensitive to touch. It had a purple/mottled color to it. It was very cold to touch. And, I was still in severe pain weeks after the injury. In early July 2008, I finally got in to see the orthopedic surgeon. This was a difficult appointment. I remember my parents went with me because they were both concerned that something wasn't right. The surgeon came in...very knowledgable, very straight forward. They whisked me off for more x-rays. When I came back, the surgeon explained that not only had I injured 4 fractures of my left foot/ankle, but I also had significant ligament damage known as a Lisfranc injury. I tore all the ligaments across my forefoot. He said that injury in and of itself would take a minimum of 1 year to heal. However, he was concerned about all these other symptoms I was showing....my foot was purple, sensitive to touch, felt like it was on fire and burned so badly, and I was still in severe pain 6 weeks after injury. I remember the doctor telling me that I was in the beginning stages of RSD/CRPS I. Due to this, I would not be able to have surgery to fix the fractures and ligament damage because the risk was too high with the RSD. RSD....RSD WHAT? I am a nurse, and I had never heard of it before. Well, come to find out, RSD is a very debilitating, progressive disease of neuropathic pain due to damage to the sympathetic nervous system that can happen after a minor injury, no injury at all, or a significant injury like what I had suffered.....those 3 letters(RSD) have changed my life forever.

There was nothing that could be done as far as the surgeon was concerned. He needed to get me into pain management to control the RSD and prevent it from spreading. However, since I was a workers comp patient, I had to wait for a C-9 approval for the consult with the pain management MD. Little did I know I would know more about workers comp and how they functioned before all was said and done. Well, because RSD did not happen immediately the day of the accident, but was a result of the injury, I had to have RSD added on as an allowed condition in my claim. Until it is added on, you can't be treated for it. I hired an attorney, knowing I was up against a fight. I put in the request for the additional allowance of RSD LLE, and sent them all of the evidence that it was RSD and was a result of the initial injury. Well, its not just that easy. It goes to a nurse, who knows she doesn't have the authority to make this decision. Then, it goes to a case manager, who also doesn't have the authority to add on a diagnosis. Then, it goes to a physician review. All they want is to deny any claims...especially RSD. Sure enough, I went in for a medical evaluation for the RSD, and the MD wrote something completely opposite. That didn't matter...my attorney knew the BWC system and hired an outside consultant to evaluate me. He wrote an 8 page consult saying what all I had been through, how delaying treatment was hurting me in the long run, etc. Then, I had to appear before the judge to get the additional allowance added on. I had so many pictures, reports, consults....how could it not be added on? Well, my attorney already prepped me and said RSD is usually not added on first try by BWC. They don't want to add that diagnosis on, because it costs them and the employer lots of money since it is a serious, chronic debilitating condition. I appeared before the judge trying not to let the tears flow.....he looked at me, looked at the evidence, and said this is a no brainer: this girl has RSD. She needs to be treated. You guys need to quit fighting it, and this condition will be allowed from this day forward. RELIEF. At least one person was on my side! I had to wait 14 days for my employer to not object to the additional allowance. They let it go through. FINALLY, I could begin treatment for my RSD. Now keep in mind the time frame.....we are now in December of 2008......I was injured May 2008. Can we say delay in treatment?

I remember my first visit with my pain management doc very vividly. He explained to me about RSD/CRPS I as best as he could. He said we needed to move fast because I was already showing signs of it spreading to my right foot. I did sympathetic nerve blocks, which helped for a few hours. He put me on med after med. This was only the beginning of a new life living on meds to control pain. I had to do rigorous physical therapy. Initially, I started in the pool and then was progressed to land therapy. After a few months, my PM doc decided that he needed to do more aggressive treatment. He wanted to place a spinal cord stimulator, which is a device that is placed in the spinal column. It has a remote that you can control the sensations down to my leg. I went through the 7 day trial....it was the first time I was pain free since the accident. Since I had a successful SCS trial, I was a candidate for permanent placement. In order to do that, I had to have a psych evaluation...a requirement by BWC. He cleared me and I agreed to obey the 12 weeks of restrictions following the surgery of no bending, twisting, turning, lifting, etc. The placement of the C-9 went through to BWC, which was approved. I had my SCS placed 2/2009.

Living with the SCS meant a few changes. I could not ride a horse, sky dive, ski, ride a wave runner, etc. I couldn't do anything that would move the leads in my back. And, as I read in the manual, I could not have children.....it was contraindicated with the SCS. Seriously??? I read it in the manual. You can't imagine how devastated I was! Trying to get over this and know how my life was changing, took a while to get used to. Each appointment I had programmers there from the company to tweak the device so that the stimulation was the best it could be to cover the pain. The SCS was amazing. It sent nice, massaging-like sensations down to my leg. This took away the pain!!!! My foot would turn normal color again, and was not sensitive to touch. I was a little less than 6 weeks post-op, and then returned to work almost a year later after the initial accident. I had mixed feelings when I returned to work. First, my employer tried to terminate me while I was off fighting for my life, if I was not back by a certain date. WHAT? Seriously? I have been fighting the BWC system to get treatment so that I can get back to work, I had all of these injuries and you are going to do what? SO, because of this threat, I was back at work a little sooner than I should have been. I was sore, no doubt, still from the surgery. I had such fear of moving equipment and doing something stupid that would move the leads in my back and ruin everything I had just been through. It took a while to get over the anger and fear of everything. I still had to go through rigorous physical therapy for over a year after the SCS placement. I was their success story. I was given less than 50% chance that I would make it back to my original position. I not only made it back to my original position as a RN, CGRN....I returned to working the same amount of hours as a full time nurse, and all the normal responsibilities that came with it. My physical therapist was amazing to get my strength back in my foot.

Over the past few years, I realized that although the SCS was helping, I would still have good days and bad days. Completely unpredictable! RSD is what it is. AND, I got so tired of trying to explain it to others, as I had enough trouble trying to understand it myself. All I know is my feet feel like they are on fire at times, and ache like crazy. They turn different colors still. Because of some increased pain with long hours, I had to cut my work hours back. This was in a way I felt like I was defeated. I always said from the beginning, I wouldn't let this RSD win. By going down in hours at work, I felt like I was letting the RSD win. But, at the same time, I had to do what was best for me. So, currently I am still a RN, CGRN working (3) 10 hr days/week.

Things started to change a few months ago. Around November or December of 2011, I started having severe spine pain in my back. It would double me over. CT Scans didn't pick up anything unusual. Doctor to doctor I went trying to find an answer. I was placed on steroids, which helped some with my RSD but not with the back pain. It wasn't until I turned my SCS off that I realized this was the cause of my back pain. The ONE thing that was truly controlling my RSD pain, was also causing me significant pain in my spine. I went to my pain management doctor, he placed me under a fluoro table and took an x-ray. This was the beginning of another nightmare....the leads had migrated 1/2 a vertebrae. This was causing ligamentous stimulation in my back, and the leads were not in the right place. WHAT??????? How could this happen? I didn't do ANYTHING that would have pulled the leads out of my back. I was beyond frustrated. My PM doc had to send me to a neurosurgeon (but, this had to be approved by BWC first). So, this started the process of having to get a revision of the SCS leads to get the SCS working again. It took weeks for the approval to go through for just a consult. I swear the people at workers comp like to make it difficult on purpose! It's a god damn consult! It was approved, thankfully. And, I got in with a neurosurgeon pretty quickly to be evaluated. Luckily, he understands the system, and his office is excellent at fighting for patients with workers comp. Currently, I am in the process of waiting for approval for a paddle lead SCS. It has more contact points on it, which allows for easier programming. They have to do a partial laminectomy(remove part of my spine) to place the lead accurately so that it doesn't move. So, this surgery will be more extensive than the initial surgery. Yes, I am scared. I know the risks involved. But, I also have to go back to remembering how much the SCS had helped me when it was truly working.

The months now that I have been waiting on approval for the SCS surgery have been pure hell. My RSD is completely out of control. I am on tons of meds, that I would not normally be on. And, I am showing early signs of spread of the RSD to my right foot/leg. I am not sleeping well at night....I wake up in severe aching/burning pain all the time. I HURT all the time. I can't even rate it on a scale of 0–10......because it doesn't fit on that scale. It is so beyond it at times,it isn't even funny. Tears just stream down my face, and I feel completely helpless at times. I am at the mercy of the BWC system for my treatment! I am still trying to maintain a normal life, which isn't quite possible at the moment. I am praying that the approval for my surgery goes through on the first try. Otherwise, my attorney will have to get involved again and do an emergency hearing.

This is my story of living with RSD. I am so young...32 years old. I should be in the prime of my life, enjoying life and all that it has to offer, yet I am right now fighting a battle to stay alive. I should have a boyfriend, but I am so scared to let anyone into my life because I would have to explain all of this to them, and I don't feel it is fair to put them through all of this. So, I remain isolated from friends. I have lost some friends over this disease, who just don't understand it and are tired of hearing me complain. My family, thank goodness, is very understanding. I don't know what I would do without my mom and dad. My poor mom has to listen to me complain all the time about hurting. As a parent, you don't want to watch your child suffer. She has been my rock, and has been keeping me going through all of this. I have a golden retriever named Bogey, who has been a life saver too. Pets know when you are in pain and at your wits end. I pray for a normal life. I pray for an answer and a cure for this monster. It absolutely ruins your life!!!!!!! I have joined support groups, which helps. I am friends with other people who have RSD, who understand what I am going through. I can see that others are worse off than me, and I also see others that have had miracles happen with a new drug called Ketamine. People have been put into remission with this drug. Unfortunately, it is not widely available and covered by insurances. I hope that in my lifetime, this ketamine treatment is something that I get to experience as it shows so much promise of putting people into remission with RSD. I hope this treatment becomes available to all of us with RSD!!!

In the meantime, I try to find my smile every day. I keep pushing forward. I continue to work, and enjoy my "new life" as much as possible. Life is too short. It took me a while to get over the anger of this whole incident. That one day that changed my life forever........such anger and so many questions why. I have to let that go and move on. Like I said, life is short. I try to remain positive. I have hope that someday there will be a cure for RSD/CRPS!!

Kerry
Certified Therapeutic Recreation Specialist

In 2000, when I was 13 years old, I was running pre-season for cross country...my FIRST year in high school!!! During a practice, I twisted my ankle, but finished the practice before finding the athletic trainer and talking with him. He told me to get an x-ray and stay off of it for a week before trying to run again.

The x-ray came back negative and I began high school on crutches, just as I was told. A week later, the pain was worse, NOT better. I went through a series of MRIs, more x-rays, bone scans, etc. Nothing was coming back with any reason as to why I was in pain. I now felt as though I was on fire, my foot was swollen, and quite discolored.

After about 3 months, my pediatrician ran out of ideas and sent me to a pediatric orthopedic about an hour away. After talking with me, my mom, and looking at my foot for about 5 minutes, he diagnosed me: Reflex Sympathetic Dystrophy. That's quite a mouthful of jumbled words with ZERO meaning for someone so young. He explained it to me that, yes, I was initially hurt and feeling pain as I should have after twisting my ankle. However, once my ankle healed, my brain was still sending pain signals to my foot, telling me that I was still hurting.

I started seeing a neurologist who had just moved into the state. He had experience working with adults with RSD and was interested to take on a pediatric. I went through months of med changes, epidurals, more meds. I remember VERY little of my freshman year due to the medication I was on. At one point, I was even using morphine lollipops! My mom, being a teacher, worked with the school to get the accommodations that I needed, including more time to finish assignments and taking exams at home with my mom sitting there with me to make sure I didn't cheat. I would only be in school a couple of hours a day, for only a couple days a week. I was taken out of school to do water therapy as it was only offered during the school day.

I was sent to Boston Children's Hospital for a week-long epidural treatment/program. Once the epidural was implanted, I walked with a PT for the first time in MONTHS. I even walked on a treadmill for .5 miles! I was EXHAUSTED after each walk, as I had lost so much muscle mass in my left leg, that I was very weak. However, towards the end of the week, the epidural shifted in my back, and the medication no longer was being sent to my leg. The RSD pains came back full-force. I had been hoping to walk out of that hospital, but instead, I was wheeled out to the car in a hospital wheelchair.

After that, my neurologist told me that the only way I would be able to walk or run again, was to just do it. I began this journey of walking again by standing with my crutches, and just touching my foot to the ground (not even any weight on it), for 10 seconds a day. Then I would put a little weight on it, then I got to the point where I could walk with crutches for a few minutes at a time. It was the most grueling of tasks, but by the end of my freshman year of high school, I was walking again, WITHOUT crutches!

By my junior year, my doctors all agreed that I could try running again. My senior year I ran on my xc team, and finished second for my team at States, and then ran the junior olympics out to New Mexico for Nationals! In college my sophomore year, my friends and I completed a half marathon! I would send my neurologist photos of each race to show him how awesome I was doing!

While training for another half marathon the following Fall, I was doing a fieldwork for a class, and a powered wheelchair ran over my RSD foot and stopped on it. Within 5 hours, I knew that I had relapsed due to the burning pain and sheer agony that I was in. My neurologist took me in the following week, and decided to do sympathetic blocks. Over a few weeks, I had two. With a change in pain meds, combined with the injections, I was back in remission by the time second semester started that year.

I graduated from UNH in 2008 in fantastic health. I got a job working in my field, and was making great new friends, and starting my life! In 2010 I started grad school for OT. This past summer, July 2011, I relapsed again, seemingly out of nowhere! The RSD has quickly spread up to my knee, and I am on a cocktail of medication. My night stand looks like a pharmacy! I have had to make the tough decision to take this Fall semester off from school to focus on my health. I struggled with this decision for a couple of weeks, but my school advisor reminded me: "you can't help other people until you help yourself." Her words are staying with me this week, as classes have begun, and I've been home trying to get better, going to PT appointments, and getting my medications changed, yet again!

I'm hopeful that the new treatments that will be starting in the next couple of months will help put me back in remission. Until then, I will keep repeating her words to myself. I can't be an effective OT if my health is terrible as well. This is the time for me to be selfish, and focus on ME and MY recovery. I think that following those words will help me to become a better OT in the future! Now is the time to help MYSELF, so I can make other people feel better.

It is a fight and a struggle every single day, to walk on a leg that feels as though it is on fire. It is a fight to focus on the end goal, through the haze of my medications. But I'm doing it. I'm fighting RSD back. This monster won't win against me...I will go into remission again!

Addendum; In September, I have gone through my first week of Ketamine infusions, and had GREAT success (the week of February 27)! I went from an 8/9 the Monday that I went in, down to a ZERO that Friday! Now that I am up and getting back to "life," the pain has increased, up to about a 3/4...but that is SO livable! I go back every 6 weeks for the remainder of the year for 3-day booster infusions. It is my hope to eventually get back to grad school, so I can become an OT, and specialize in working with patients with RSD!
--
 Tell me and I forget, teach me and I remember, involve me and I learn. – Benjamin Franklin

My story
By Mary

I was heading towards the end of 7th grade, it was either April or May (can't remember which). I had just finished the middle school musical (School House Rock Live Jr.) and had a role as a ensemble member, but had a solo in one of the songs. I was never athletic, but played the violin and sang. However, my elementary school was across the street with basketball courts. A friend and I were shooting hoops and talking about how the year was almost over and our summer plans. Suddenly I tripped over my left foot and it went sideways. Two days later it still hurt so my mom took me to the pediatrician. He said oh she doesn't walk right, so take her to a podiatrist. My mom and i thought that was the wrong specialist to go to and since our insurance doesn't require referrals for specialists, my mom decided to make me an appointment with Temple Sports Medicine. The doctor there took an x-ray and didn't see anything in the x-ray but said a lot of times stress fractures won't show and that's what he suspected I had. He put me in a walking boot. I saw him a month or two later and this time I was still in pain and it had spread to my hands as well. He ordered blood work suspecting juvenile arthritis and a bone scan to see if there was a stress fracture still present. In the mean time I was to continue in the boot. The bone scan was normal,but the blood work showed a positive ANA. He recommended that I go see a rheumatologist. At the time i was young, so I couldn't see any of the rheumatologist he knew cause they would only see 18+. I went to CHOP (Children's Hospital of Philadelphia). In the mean time i started doing some research on positive ANA's with my mom. I was convinced I had either Arthritis or Lupus. The doctor there knew I had RSD (but they called it RND) right away because Dr. David Sherry worked there. They said i would have to be in Dr. Sherry's program of PT /OT and it would be rough and how they see kids crying in the hallway doing it but it works. My mom asked if I could do the program with any PT and she said no. I was crying because as I said I was never physical and I thought great if I couldn't' be active before how can I do it now when I'm in pain? I was enrolled in the program from Halloween to the day before Thanksgiving of my 8th grade year. By that point I couldn't turn the dial of my locker. The program was hell. It helped a lot though.

By high school and in high school i was at an average of a 0-4 pain level daily. Then Junior year i went to prom. Late that night my foot hurt, but I thought oh maybe its from dancing too much. But the pain never went away and it got worse. From then on my pain kept getting worse. It was manageable senior year and most of my freshman year of college. But the end of freshman year of college my new rheumatologist who I had been seeing for carpal and cubital tunnel sent me to Dr. Schwartzman that summer. She had gotten me in so quickly because she works for Drexel as well. He recommended ketamine but said I would have to be off my anti depressant meds and I couldn't do that plus insurance wouldn't cover it. Then we found Cooper Pain Management and my first appointment was July 28th of that summer (the day after my 20th birthday). I soon had 6 nerve blocks which helped initially but not towards the end. I had three day continuous epidural over my winter break in the hospital. It helped a bit but not enough. And the pain returned. I tired some outpatient ketamine, but it wasn't as helpful as hoped. I even tried an epidural injection. The last few months of my sophomore year of college were the worst. I rarely attended class, i almost quit. This summer i have spent most of it in bed. After having RSD for 8 years now, I hadn't been to the ER for RSD ever, but in 2012 I went 4 times. The one time I went to the hospital my doctor works for they did pretty much nothing and treated me like a drug addict/seeker. They had the fact that il had RSD on record but ignored it. They finally after begging gave me a script for a few perocet but wouldn't give me one at the time when I was in agony and it was too late that night to go to the pharmacy and get one unless I went to a 24 hour one where they didn't have my insurance info.

I've been to one calmare consult (to be explained in Emily's Story) and it was very helpful. I'm trying calmare for ten more sessions July 9–19th everyday but Sunday. I'm hoping for the best.

RSD has changed my life. I can no longer make and keep plans as often as I'd like with friends because i always end up having to cancel due to pain flares. People get mad at me for being unreliable and I used to be a reliable person.

Rachel Anne McLoud's RSD Story

I have had problems with pain for most of my life. I remember being eight years old and having to ride in my little brother's stroller because my legs were hurting for a reason that no one could explain. Thankfully, my mother has always believed me when I have told her that I was in pain; even when there was no physical evidence to back up my claims. These pains when I was young came and went. They were mysterious but they never lasted very long. I had a fairly normal childhood until I was thirteen.

At thirteen a series of three small injuries compiled themselves into one big problem. First, I was babysitting and I wrenched my knee on a swing (I was a very clumsy kid). Next, even though I was sore, I went rollerskating and fell on the same knee. Finally, and most significantly, I slipped UP the stairs. My mother was recovering from gallbladder surgery, so I was doing the laundry for her. While carrying a laundry basket and wearing socks on carpeted stairs, (none of these smart decisions) I slipped going up the stairs. I only slid down three stairs, but that was enough to injure the already hurt right knee.

I first went to my general doctor. He said it was a minor sprain and advised that I wrap it in an Ace bandage. He gave me some crutches and sent me on my way. Two weeks later, I was still in pain. I went to another doctor. This doctor decided it was a much more severe sprain, put me in a full leg brace for a month and left me on the crutches. I was now known as "Crip" at school. After a month I was still in pain.

I went to an Orthopedic Surgeon. We did our research and found the best in the city. He was actually the sports doctor for the Atlanta Braves. He did an exam and decided that I had a nasty sprain that wasn't healing properly because it had been in the brace too long. He sent me to physical therapy. (One interesting side note. Many years later after I had gotten the diagnosis of RSD I went back to this doctor and asked for a transcript of my medical history. In his notes from my first exam he had written, "might possibly be RSD." !!! He never said a word. Never. I went years in his practice as I will explain and he never once suggested RSD!)

I went to his physical therapist. He was horrified that I had been in the brace for over a month. Apparently, if I had been in for a week or two more, I would have been in danger or losing the use of my leg permanently. Nice doctors I was seeing! Anyway, the therapist I saw was terrific. He worked me hard. He used to compare me to the grunting ballplayers who were complaining next to me and say, "this little girl is doing twice what you're doing and not saying a word, so shut up!" I met a lot of the top athletes of the time at that office. It was fun! When I had to have cortisone shots under my kneecap, these huge men would turn white, thinking it was for them, and the doctor would have to show them that it was being given to a little 13 year-old to shame them. It would encourage me to not make a sound when I was given the shots.

After months of treatment with the therapist, plus regular cortisone shots, I wasn't getting any better. I was still in pain. I had had several X-rays and MRIs but nothing had shown up in any of the scans. I even had something called an arthrogram. They inject dye and air into the the affected joint and then scan it. It's not used very much today. It hurt like hell. It was funny afterward though. Every time I moved, the air in my knee sounded like squishing Jello between my teeth!

Finally the only option was exploratory orthoscopic surgery. I was fourteen. I had been on crutches for over a year now, so it was a no-brainer. I had the surgery and once inside they found a very small tear in my cartilage and a small nick on my ligament. The doctor repaired them. He said he was puzzled though because such small injuries shouldn't have caused me so much pain.

Following surgery I was put into heavy-duty physical therapy. It included TENS therapy which helped a lot. After a month I was back to my old self again. I was relatively pain-free and healthy. I occasionally had days where I had some pain. I attributed it to having had surgery. But for the most part, I had a normal life. I hiked, rock-climbed, mountain biked, danced and lived a very active life.

I graduated and went to art school. It was a very intense course. I was taking more classes than normal and extra-long studio classes. I'm an over-achiever by nature and getting "A's" is the only option for me. I was getting up early and going to bed very, very late. I would stay at school until the building closed because I didn't own my own computer and I needed to work on the school's computers. I was also holding down a high pressure internship and working on the weekends. I have a rich spiritual life as well and I didn't allow that to suffer. Needless to say, I was stressed out. I had little time to rest.

This was 1996 and the Olympics were in town. I was 21. I happened to have a free afternoon and my best friend and I wanted to see the "Rings" exhibit of the masterworks that were in town because of the Olympics. She was an art student as well. We walked all over the exhibit looking at the art. Afterward we walked all around the Olympic Village and around the city. It was a terrific day. I remember it so clearly. I even remember what I was wearing, because the next morning I woke up and I couldn't walk.

I was in excruciating pain. This time it was in both knees. And the unusual thing was the left knee, the one I hadn't previously injured or had surgery on, hurt more. (That's still the case, by the way. The left is always worse than the right. Weird!) I didn't understand what was going on. I tried to remember if I had fallen or hurt myself the day before, but nothing came to mind. All I had done the day before was walk around. Now I couldn't even move without searing pain shooting through my body and in both knees.

I went back to the orthopedic surgeon. He checked both legs and there was nothing physically wrong with either leg. He couldn't give me a reason for why I was in such pain or why it was in both legs. (Again, why he didn't suggest RSD, I will never know.)

Then began my odyssey into the medical community. I saw doctor after doctor. One doctor told me I should become a ballerina, that that would fix my problems (?!). Another told me that I should do the Marines workout everyday, that that would ease my pain. More than a few told me that the pain was all in my head. One doctor took a reflex hammer and hit my knee so hard tears ran down my cheeks and I screamed. Then, he started to do the other one! I grabbed the hammer out of his hand before he could do it. I said, "if the first one hurt that much, let's just suppose that the other one will too, okay?" I did see a few nice doctors, but even they couldn't tell me what was wrong with me. I must say at this point that my parents never once doubted that there was something wrong with me and they never doubted that we would find out what was wrong, even though I did.

Finally one doctor who specialized in arthritis suggested that I see a doctor named Sam Schatten. (It's funny, I've seen so many doctors in my life that I've forgotten most of their names, even the ones I saw for years. But I will never forget his name. He is the man that gave a name to my pain.) He specialized in diagnosing diseases that no one else could. He was sort of a real Dr. House except that he doesn't treat the disease, he only diagnoses it. So we looked him up and went to see him.

Dr. Schatten is one of the strangest people I have ever met in my life. If he doesn't have O.C.D. I would be shocked. He spent over three hours with me. I think he only touched me three times. But he asked hundreds of questions – questions that none of the other doctors had ever thought to ask me: did my skin change color? was it cold or warm? had I noticed any changes in the hair? describe the pain in as much detail as possible. The whole time he was asking these questions he was buzzing around the room. He would arrange papers. He lined up his books with a ruler, like ten times! He paced. I'm assuming it's just part of his process. After three hours, he suddenly snapped his fingers and said, "I know what you have!" He ran out of the room and didn't come back for fifteen minutes. My mom, dad and I just stared at each other and wondered, "was this guy nuts?" When he came back he was holding a large medical text that I assume he had gotten from another library (the room that we were in housed a fair amount of medical texts as well). He began to recite the symptoms of RSD. They lined up perfectly with what I had.

It was like a giant weight was suddenly lifted from my shoulders. It had a name! I wasn't crazy! You see, even though I knew the pain was real, I had a lot of doubts myself. I had seen so many doctors, had so many tests that had come up with no answers, I was beginning to think that maybe it really was all in my head. Maybe I was experiencing the normal aches and pains that everyone feels and I was just a drama queen. It's hard to doubt professionals that have gone to school for medicine when they're telling you you're crazy! But finally, here was a doctor telling me that not only did I have a disease, but that it had a name and that it had been around since the Civil War. My next question to him was, how do I fight this? He said, "Sorry kid, that's not my department. That's going to be your job from now on." I left his office with a bizarre mixture of worry and relief.

I took a leave of absence from school and from my internship and took on the job of fighting my illness full-time. We found a doctor in Canton, GA, which is about an hour and a half away from my house, that could treat me. First he gave me a nerve block to make sure that the diagnosis of RSD was certain. I was sedated and the block was done, targeting my knees. When I woke up, the first thing I felt was warm feet and warm knees for the first time in months. One of the side effects of RSD is the narrowing of the blood vessels to prevent me from bleeding to death from my tragic injury (yeah, right!). The block tricked the nerves and the vessels opened flooding my knees with blood for the first time in ages. It felt sooo good! (Oddly, when my knees are really bad, my feet get cold as well. I can always tell how bad my knees are going to be by how cold my feet are.)

After the certain diagnosis, we started on treatment. I first started with a drug regimen. When that didn't do much my doctor discussed more intense options. First we tried a series of nerve blocks every few weeks. They would work for a few days but would wear off quickly. I was young and anxious to get on with my life. My doctor decided something more aggressive was needed. He suggested an epidural catheter. It would be dosed every day so that I could get the pain relief that I needed and be able to do the physical therapy that was so critical to getting the disease into remission. I agreed and the catheter was implanted. I would get up very early in the morning and drive to Canton and get dosed. Then, we would drive to the city to my physical therapist for an hour and a half of intense therapy, then home to crash. I was sick most of those mornings. I have a weak stomach anyway and mornings and I rarely agree. I think I saw more of the road shoulders of Georgia and Atlanta than most highway workers do. I really don't know how my mother did it – chauffeuring me through that month. She is my angel on earth. Anyway, we did this for a month, including weekends. I bathed in two inches of water so as not to get the catheter infected. It was a difficult month to say the least. But a month after this treatment I was in remission. I still walked a little slowly but I was definitely recovered. Looking back I accredit this treatment working so well because we caught the disease fairly early and treated it very aggressively, very quickly. I am really grateful for that.

I went back and finished school and got my degree. I got a

job in publishing as a graphic designer. I moved out into my own apartment. I had a nice life. It wasn't the most thrilling life, but it was fun. I went dancing on the weekends. I got back into rock climbing and biking and hiking. I was very social. But then my over-achiever personality reared it's ugly head. I eventually became an art director of a small magazine. I started working ridiculous hours. I would get up fairly early and stay at work until very, very late. My job came with a lot of stress. I wasn't eating well or taking care of myself very well. Looking back on it I wish I could shake myself and just say, "NO! What are you doing?!" Especially since it was exactly what had caused me to get sick the first time around, you think I would know better. But I didn't.

This time it started slowly. After my college sickness, I would occasionally have a sore day here or there. I would walk with a cane that day, but the next day it would be over. I didn't really think much of it. So when I had a couple of pain days in a row, I didn't think it was such a big deal. But then a couple of days turned into a week. And then two weeks. Then a month. Then I had to start using crutches. Finally I had to stop lying to myself – the pain was back. My bosses knew about my illness. I started working from home and telecommuting when I could, but they weren't too happy about it (the company had recently changed hands and my nice boss had been replaced with a total jerk). I had to come in later and later in the day because mornings were harder and harder, but I would always stay late enough to make it an eight hour day and I always made sure that my work was done and that my clients were happy. I started to have to use a wheelchair. My bosses offered me a new position on the swing shift. I decided to take it. Then, out of the blue, they decided to eliminate this position instead of giving it to me. I opted to quit before they could fire me.

I had reached my breaking point. I could no longer take care of myself. I went to my parents and asked for help. I asked if I could move home for a few months. They knew about my job situation. They were so kind and so supportive. (Not so my roommate even though I was still paying rent, but I won't bore you with that story!) I moved back into my childhood bedroom and started over in my fight against pain.

I decided not to go back to my previous doctor because of the drive time. We did some research and found a pain clinic much closer to home. There I found the most amazing doctor. The first time I went to his practice, I almost walked out before I saw him. I waited four and a half hours to see him! It turned out to be worth the wait. He runs behind schedule all of the time because he takes so much time with each patient. He was kind and gentle, personable and funny. It was like meeting a long-lost friend. I found out that he was an insatiable researcher. He always wanted to be on the cusp of technological and medical advances. I was his willing guinea pig. I tried every drug and every device. Everything was met with varying degrees of success. Most of the drugs made me sick as a dog. But I have learned that my body eventually adapts to just about anything.

In 2000 I had my first spinal cord stimulator implanted. First they did the test with leads that were outside of my body. The results were amazing! I had no pain for the first time in years. I immediately wanted the surgery. I had one of the old, non-rechargeable versions, which meant that I had to have the battery changed surgically. I was running the unit at full blast on both leads to cover both knees. That meant that I ran my batteries out really fast – about nine months time. I started having surgery every nine months for the next three years.

After I recovered from the first implantation, I felt so good that I decided that I wanted to come off of all of my medication. At the time I was on about 600 milligrams of Methadone, not to mention Oxycodone for breakthrough pain. My doctor prescribed Subutex to help me step down on the Methadone. Despite that, it was the most awful hell I have ever experienced in my life. I have never been so sick. It took three months to come off of all of the medications. By the time I came off of everything, my brain had started to figure out the workings of the stimulator and the pain was starting to creep back. Go figure.

By the time I was ready for my fourth stimulator, Medtronic had made a rechargeable one. Unfortunately, had I been able to wait just two months more, I would have had the stimulator that's the size of a quarter and charges in fifteen minutes. Mine is the size of an old-school IPod and charges in five hours. You have to be tethered to a wall outlet to charge. Did I mention where the stim is located? Let's just say that I sit on it all the time. Not that comfortable. I can't get the new one until the old one dies. Ah well, my luck. J

You may be thinking, this girl has some fabulous insurance to be getting all these stimulators! Well, after I quit my job, I started the long process of getting disability. It was very difficult. The first time I applied I was turned down because I was apparently too young to be disabled (?!). The next time I was too educated. You only get three chances. So I got a lawyer. On the third go-round I went before a judge. I don't remember much about that day except for one question that was asked of me. It was really more of a statement, actually. The judge said, "You don't really look that sick to me." I thanked her and told her that I work very hard at not looking sick. I disguise my grey skin with makeup. I also hide my purple knees with clothing or makeup. And I try to always have a cheerful, sunny disposition, because I don't want to be known and The Sick Girl, or the 'girl with the disease', I just want to be The Girl. She granted my application that day. Medicare has been a godsend. I wouldn't be able to pay for any of the medical procedures that I've had done without it. I also have gap insurance that takes care of the rest. It's expensive. Disability doesn't actually pay much. If I wasn't able to live at home, I would probably be homeless. I don't know how some people do it. I makes me really sympathize with people in situations harder than my own. And I can see how you could easily get underwater very fast with a chronic illness.

A few years ago my dear, sweet doctor became ill himself. He developed cancer and had to turn his practice over to his partner. His partner is also a very nice man, though not as involved as he was. I recently thought it over and realized that I had each doctor when I really needed them most, though. The first was the hand-holding sort and that's what I really needed when I was just coming to grips with the grief of losing my former life. My current doctor is kind of a "wham-bam-thank-you-ma'am" type, and that's cool for now because I'm comfortable with my situation now. I don't need the hand-holding anymore. I can stand on my own two feet now.

The stimulator high didn't last forever and I eventually had to go back on medication. I'm back on the Methadone, and ironically, it's a higher dose than before. I still use the stimulator. On the pain scale it takes off about 1.5 - 2 notches of pain, so it's worth using. I know the minute it "dies" and can't wait until it charges!

I am now getting regular Ketamine treatments. I get them once a month, two days in a row. At first they were the most hellish thing I had ever experienced. The hallucinations were unbearable! I won't describe them, because I can barely understand them myself. I would literally scream at the top of my lungs for most of the five hour treatment. It was understandably a little disconcerting for the other patients in the clinic. I would try to jump out of bed or hit the nurses and my mother. It was awful. Finally they found out that by giving me a dose of Versed every twenty minutes, I would stay calm. If they were even one minute late, the screaming would start. Then, a few months ago the doctor's office called to tell me that there was a nationwide shortage of Versed and that they wouldn't be able to give me my treatment with it. I was terrified. There was no way that I could do it without the Versed, but I needed my treatment to keep the pain at a bearable level. They suggested that I try the treatment with an infusion of Propofol. They would give me enough to sedate me, but not enough to put me to sleep and they would have someone watching me the whole time. I agreed because I really had no other choice. Thank goodness I did! The Propofol was a revelation! I ended up sleeping through my entire treatment – something I had never done before. I hadn't had a single hallucination and the bonus was it left my system much quicker than the Versed, so I was much less groggy afterward. Ever since then, that has been my routine. On my last visit, they added an infusion of Lidocaine to the mix and that added an extra amount of pain relief. It was just something to try and it really worked well.

I have very small veins that collapse very easily. The Ketamine treatments require an I.V. to be put in every time. So I was having an I.V. put in once a month and I was quickly running out of veins, because once a vein was used it could never be used again. Also, since I go for two days in a row the I.V. has to last for both days. Often it would get inflamed because the vein was just too small to handle it. About five months ago I had a sub-clavian port put in and it is the best thing I've done in a while. It is so much easier to get the lines put in. The surgery was very simple. I've added to my collection of scars, but I've resigned myself to being the Patchwork Girl!

I'm always game to try something new because you never know what might work. I've tried just about everything under the sun in the hopes that it just might work. I've tried all manner of 'natural' and homeopathic techniques. I've tried herbs. I've tried Eastern medicines. Acupuncture. Sound therapy. I actually own a hyperbaric chamber. I does work a little bit, but it takes the dedication of getting in it every day. Betar tables. Special diets. Exercise regimens. I've taken every drug there is to take. There are a few new things out that I can't try now that I have the stimulator because of the radio waves, but other than that, you name it, I've tried it.

I'm a surprisingly content person. Most people are surprised to find that out about me. Yes, large parts of my life royally suck, but there are so many good parts that I try to concentrate on them and let them overshadow the bad. I try really hard to keep a good attitude and keep a smile on my face. Nobody wants to be around a complaining mope. That's not to say that I don't have my bad days. I allow myself a pity party every now and again. But I don't let myself wallow. I decided a long time ago that whining was not an option and that I wasn't going to let this disease break my spirit.

I did have one really dark period early in my college bout. I got really depressed and couldn't get out of it. Nothing seemed to work. I just didn't want to keep going. Nothing seemed to matter anymore. One night I decided that I was just going to take whatever pills I had in my cabinet and be done with it. That night my friend was dropping me off. He had no idea what was going on in my head. Suddenly he turned to me and said, "You know, there are a lot of people who really love you and would miss you if you weren't here." I just stared at him, goosebumps all over my arms. He just turned and walked away. It was totally unlike him to say something like that, too. That night I told my mom what I had been planning and asked her to keep my pills with her until I was in a better frame of mind. I never thought about suicide again. After that experience I tried to focus on the other people in my life instead of turning inward like I had been doing.

I attribute a lot of my successful good attitude to my spiritual life. I'm one of Jehovah's Witnesses and my faith is my life. My relationship with God is everything. Because I've had to rely on Him so much, my relationship with him has gotten so much closer. I always say, it's the one good thing that you can get out of chronic illness. I draw so much strength and comfort from prayer and from reading the Bible and spiritual literature. And I look forward to the paradise earth that is promised in the Bible where "no resident will say, 'I am sick'". (Isaiah 33:24)

As I have mentioned throughout this, well, what is now a treatise (sorry!), my family has been amazingly supportive of me. My dad is my fixer. Whenever a problem comes up, he says, "okay, how are we going to tackle this one?" He loves to research new ways to treat my disease. He is so confident that I am going to be in remission again one day. My mom is my comfort and my best friend. She has some nerve pain herself so she can commiserate and empathize. Mom is also my primary care-giver. She helps me clean my apartment (I have a small apartment in my parent's basement, now), she drives me everywhere I need to go, she does my grocery shopping for me, and she is my medical advocate. I don't know what I'd do without her. I also have a brother and sister-in-law. They are my cheerleaders. They get so excited any time I can do anything other than my usual day-to-day stuff. They push me to do more and are so proud when I can. I lost a lot of friends when I got sick. A lot of people just weren't up to the challenge. But the people who stick around are the ones that you want to keep, anyway. I have amazing friends. They are so understanding when I have to cancel last-minute because I made plans, but I'm having a bad pain day. They're so helpful when we're at a party and I can't balance a plate of food and my cane and a flight of stairs. And they never make me feel that it's any big deal; that I'm anything less than normal. Everyone should be so lucky as to have friends like mine.

So I think that's it. I'm pretty sure I gave you a lot more than you wanted, but once I got started it was hard to stop. As I said before, feel free to edit as you see fit. I hope this helps you and maybe can help some other people too. All we have are each other's experiences and the more we lean on each other the stronger we are.

Melissa's story
October 14th 2009,11 days after my wedding, my sister and I decided to go to Walmart with my son to buy him some new pajamas to wear at grandma's house while we were on our honeymoon. There was a door greeter at Walmart sitting in his wheelchair that had these cute pumpkin wheel covers. My sister and I were talking about them. There was a group of people standing in front of the buggies blocking the way so my sister took my son and went ahead in the store. I grabbed the buggy and went to meet her.

I was putting my purse in my buggy when all of a sudden I was run over with the door greeter in his wheelchair. He was backing up and ran over my ankle. Not thinking anything about it I thought no big deal it hurts. It was just like stubbing your toe I'll be okay. Later that night we went home and I propped and iced my foot like you would do with any other normal minor injury. The next day it was still hurting and actually gotten worse. It started swelling even more and turning black and blue. I called the people at Walmart to notify them what'd happen. Later that day I went to the ER with a took x-rays and told me nothing was wrong. It was just a sprained ankle. They gave me a ankle brace and crutches and sent me out the door. I left for my honeymoon 2 days later after my grandmother's wedding wearing an air brace on a pair of crutches. Luckily the church I worked at loaned me a wheelchair for our honeymoon so I wouldn't have to be on crutches for the whole week. My ankle was still hurting when I got back so I went to see my doctor. He referred me to the orthopedic.That orthopedic specialists took a look at my leg and ankle and then sent me to physical therapy and prescribed lyrica. I had an allergic reaction to it. After a month of physical therapy it was no help so the doctor referred me to a specialist for ankle and foot. He even had an MRI. He took a look at that there was nothing wrong with me. He then gave me a cortisone injection as well as steroids,and tramodol. He placed me in a walking boot for a little bit and told me that I probably just tore some ligaments and it might take up to 6 months for it to heal.But after 6 months then he decided that he thought I might have lupus so he sent me to a rheumatologist to have me tested for lupus arthritis and fibromyalgia. when I got to the rheumatologist he looked at me and laughed and said I don't know why you're even here, your symptoms match anything I do. I tell you everything came back fine you just have low vitamin D.

I went back to my regular doctor and then he referred me to a different orthopedic group. That doctor look at all the other medical records from the other two and ordered another x-ray and another MRI. He also scheduled a series of blocks to be performed by the pain specialist and told me that I have complex regional pain syndrome. I was freaking out not knowing what was going to happen to me. After going home and looking this up he then told me that the pain doctor would call me to setup the blocks. So I got to the pain specialist and setup my appointment. I explain to him that I have a needle phobia and then I have to be knocked out for anything that would involve a needle. He agreed. When I got there for the blocks the doctor decided to tell me that they were not going to put me out. That they were just going to give me a pill that would calm down my nerves. Then I would just go with it and have the procedure done. I started freaking out and hyperventilating. Then they agreed to knock me out completely. After the block I was headed home and the pain was still there yet I would need to come back and have the second block done at two weeks. When I returned the second time I told them that it did nothing for me the first time. They again said that they would not knock me out. I started freaking out hyperventilating again. They agreed to knock me out because I was hyperventilating and freaking out. They didn't give me a small dose of the twilight because it took longer for it to work then normal. They accuse me of being a drug addict. When the test came back clean they told me to seek therapy because no one could be this afraid of needles. Once I had gotten my needle phobia taking care of then I can come back and get the rest of my blocks. I went back to my ortho doctor who had scheduled the block and explain to him what it happen. He sent me another pain management specialist. The new doctors office call and ordered a bone scan then they offered to give me a spinal cord simulator but I did not want it. They explain to me that that was there only option because I have a lot of allergies to narcotics as well as meds like lyrica. The ortho doctor sent me back to a physical therapy again to see if it would work now but after 3 months of no improvement. They gave me a 10 minute a list of exercises and a Tens unit to do at home. The TENS seem to make everything worse instead of making it better. I felt alone and unsure of what to do. I went on Facebook looking to find some support to see if I could find someone who had this same crazy thing that I'd never even heard of. Because of Facebook I found a wonderful new list treatment options that were out there that I had to search for. Because I just had a baby I need to make sure that I can do whatever and still breastfeed. I had it down to either hyper barrack oxygen therapy or ketatine infusions. I looked all around Nashville and couldn't find anything near me but I did find a doctor in Jackson TN who did HBOT. It was four thousand dollars. He told me that if bumped my foot too hard I would have to start all over because it would return and I would no longer be in remission. He added that insurance wouldn't cover it. I found a doctor in Atlanta that offer Ketamine infusions . My insurance covered it so we picked Ketamine. It was the best choice I made. I have my life back well as much as possible. I'm not lying in the bed sleeping and crying wishing that a bus would hit me.

My son was 4 when I got hurt and its hard to explain to a child that young why mommy can't take him to the zoo whenever he wants and why I can't climb down in the floor to play cars and trains anymore. His funny exciting free sprit mom has been replaced by a stressed, depressed, and overly careful mother. Here he is now seven and he asks me every time I go to the doctor if my foot is fixed and all better. He tells me all the time I love you mom but I miss the old you. Went are you going to be like that again? I know its that same feeling that kids with divorced parents get where they always hope that will get back together. Its sad and makes me feel guilty and that's a hard feeling to knock. Its been three years now Me and my family are trying to get use to the new normal and its always changing but were are hanging in there on this roller coaster of emotional.

12-12-12
By Alexia

So how does a woman explain how she acquired RSD? Is there a special protocol that must be followed to lay the proper groundwork or to pique the interest of your desired audience? I don't know. I do think it requires the author to be straight-forward and not worry about who might understand your desire to turn your most intimate thoughts, feelings, and craziness into your personal journey. I have always believed that life is messy, challenging and full of moments of great learning, insight, love and soul-searching. Living with an auto-immune disease such as RSD makes life even more so.

Before I can reveal the details surrounding my twelve years of living with RSD, I must share with you what happened on July 14, 2009, a seemingly normal hot day in Frisco, Texas. Little did I know that a freak home accident would change the rest of my life forever, revealing an unruly child called RSD had entered my life many years earlier and slammed its wicked door in my face while I was fighting for my life.

But I am getting ahead of myself so let me get back on track. It was spring of 2009 and my husband Michael told me that he needed a new suitcase for his work travel. After searching off and on for a couple of weeks, he still hadn't purchased a new one (this one is too big, this one is too small, this one is too expensive, this one will fall apart too quickly.....on and on). So in hopes to end the search, our sons and I decided to help him find a new suitcase. Lo and behold we finally succeeded. In June, my parents came out from CA and stayed a couple of weeks and, as they always do, they put their suitcases in our master bedroom along the left wall. Just before they went home, Michael had to leave town and came home about one week later. It is customary for me to "air out" his suitcase when he gets home because his closed-up suitcase with both clean and dirty clothing usually ends up with that distinctive odor of only dirty clothing. So after he unpacked it, I moved it to where my parents' suitcases had been, opened it up and sprayed some deodorizing spray. Not thinking more about it, I was doing laundry two days later and after emptying our dryer and walking into our bedroom, I walked right into the suitcase. Okay, "walked" isn't the right word.....I literally slammed my left foot right into the side of the suitcase. My pinky toe received the brunt of the slam and I did the normal song and dance one does when this type of thing occurs. But being the kind of woman I am, I brushed it off as a bad stubbing of my toe, folded the laundry and went on my day. Our sons and I went to our community pool later that afternoon and saw my good friend Teresa there. As I was telling her about the accident, I realized that my entire left foot did not like being in the nice warm water. That night, I took a shower, gingerly put some lotion on my feet, put on some socks and went to bed. All night, I was aware that this toe and the entire left side of my left foot were talking to me, but I did my best to ignore it and tried to sleep.

The next morning, I was horrified to take off my socks and discover that my pinky toe and some of the left side of my foot was literally purple. I called my internist and explained what happened and we concluded that I must have broken my toe. Ice it, elevate it, take some ibuprofen, stay off it and call if I don't feel better in a couple of days. I did just that, feeling completely foolish about the entire thing. Michael teased me for moving and airing out his suitcase, then decided it was a good idea to put it away in our walk-in closet. After all, you can't have an idiot like me walking around in our bedroom with a suitcase on the floor; I might just do it again!

By that Friday, I was feeling even more foolish when I realized that instead of feeling better, my toe and foot felt much worse. I promptly phoned my internist again and she told me to come in for x-rays. Sure enough the damage was clear and it was possible that I even dislocated my toe. After a quick referral to an orthopedist that unfortunately couldn't see me until Monday morning, I was sent home again to continue the ice/elevation/ibuprofen routine.

Monday morning couldn't come soon enough and the x-rays were repeated. In his opinion, I didn't dislocate my toe but I broke it in two places and he put me in a sandal-like soft boot. Yes, continue with the ice/elevation/ibuprofen routine. I continued to see him over the course of a few weeks and noticed that even though my toe was no longer purple, my ankle and foot were huge and I had intense burning coming from the pinky toe, the toe immediately next to it and the entire left side of my foot. As time went by, the burning and pain crossed to all my toes, to my ankle and was now shooting up my leg to my hip. It was like someone was lighting a firework from my toe to my hip and then it would go off. By now my breaks have healed, parts of my left foot were either numb or burning and the orthopedist is annoyed that I am having all this pain. Oh, I must not be doing the home exercises correctly or I'm not icing it enough (which was true because now my foot can't stand the ice therapy anymore) or frankly I am just bitching. Finally he gives me the name and phone number of a pain management specialist and tells me that if I don't feel "better" after a month, to come back.

After realizing that this doctor wants me gone, gone, gone (and just maybe the door will hit my ass on the way out!), I agree with my mom (who's an RN and an auto-immune sufferer herself) to see a neurologist. I call a girlfriend who is seeing a neurologist for her auto-immune disorder and make an appointment to get a second opinion. This lovely female neurologist is sympathetic, warm and frankly a bit horrified that not only was my foot not cast for the break, but that I hadn't actually been directly referred to a neurologist when it was clear that not only did my nerve pain never go away, but only intensified as the weeks went by. She immediately puts me on some medication which makes me incredibly loopy and eventually conducts an EMG. After reviewing the results, she is hopeful that the foot surgeon next door can help me and sends the results of my EMG to her. My hope that a foot surgery will solve my problem, however, is dashed when the surgeon runs a nerve block test on my left leg and rather than feeling relief, my pain increases. She has me purchase an Aircast FP Walker from her office assistant, orders an MRI of my foot and tells me to bring the CD of the images to my next visit. After reviewing the images and discussing my case with her colleague, the surgeon tells me that she knows exactly what is wrong with me and surgery will not solve the problem. I am diagnosed with RSD. Stoically, I take the news and I am given the name and contact information of a pain management doctor who specializes in RSD. I am asked to give her the MRI CD and make an appointment immediately. I reach my car, shut the door and begin to sob. I phone

Michael who is at work and he tells me that he will leave work and come home. I call my Mom and both of us cry. She stays on the line till I pull into my driveway and wait for Michael to get home. I feel like Hell has walked into my life and it wears a chain around my neck called RSD.

I have been a patient of Dr. Elizabeth Eversull's now for a few months. My labs have been all over the place. Some medications agree with me and others don't. Elizabeth is kind, patient and clearly worried. She has asked me to come in a day early to discuss my latest lab results.

Elizabeth comes into the exam room with my chart and several pieces of paper. She sits down directly across from me and uses the examination table that sits in the middle of the room as a desk. She asks me to pull up my chair to the table. She leans forward and puts her hands on the paperwork and looks me directly in the eye. She tells me that she needs to ask me a very important question and she apologizes for asking it because it is not normally a question someone asks another. I tell her to come out with it......ask it. She takes a deep breath and asks me if I have ever had a near-death experience.

Although the question surprises me, the way Elizabeth is looking at me you would think she asked me if I had led some "secret past" involving the mob. I answer "yes" and she looks both relieved and upset all at the same time. She asks me what happened and I tell her. She says it explains EVERYTHING.....the pieces of the puzzle is now coming together. This is my story:

In 1997 I was 29 years old. I had never been married and had no children. For many years I tremendously enjoyed my single life by attending college, traveling alone and with friends, living on my own, writing poetry and short stories (with some of them published in the United States, England and Australia), working various jobs and dating, dating, dating. Many of my friends who had already married were either divorced within a couple of years or were still married but miserable. Some of them were already on a second marriage and others had sworn off marriage altogether. So needless to say, I was very leery of getting married.

A friend of mine suggested that join a "chat site" that had nothing to do with dating; it was a "pen pal" site dedicated to making friends around the world sans the snail mail process. It seemed like a fun idea so I signed up and entered the site. After being online for just a few minutes, a "Michael" from South Africa came online. Michael was considered one of the original members of the site "family" because he had been on that site since it began. But none of that mattered to me; by the end of our "introduction" on the site, I knew that somehow, some way, Michael and I would be married. I can't explain even today how or why I knew this; I just did.

Within a matter of months, we had exchanged photographs, were openly discussing our feelings for one another and then began chatting on the phone. By this time, we had chatted almost everyday on this site plus we were sending each other pages and pages of emails. Then during one conversation, Michael asked me if I could come to South Africa for the Christmas holiday. Originally Michael thought that here in the States, we had the same three week holiday "break" that they had in South Africa. When we discuss the cost of the airfare and the amount of time I would have to take off work to be in South Africa during this break, I simply told Michael that if I went to South Africa, I wouldn't just do it as a trip. After a pause, Michael told me that if I flew out to South Africa, he would want me to stay. So when I asked him what he meant by that, he told me that if I flew to South Africa, he would want me to stay and have us get married. It may have been an awkward marriage proposal, but considering the circumstances, nothing about our relationship was conventional. I immediately said yes and then wondered how in the world we could make this happen.

As it turned out, I flew out the day after Thanksgiving in 1997. Although I was now 30 years old, it is putting it mildly that some of my friends and my family thought I was completely crazy and concerned for my safety. Others however were caught up in the "romance" of it all and how old-fashioned in some ways it seemed; rather than developing our relationship on looks and material things, it was developed on conversations, emails and chatting. I asked my family to have faith in my decision and with great hesitation, they did.

Some people might have thought that I would come home in a matter of days with my tail between my legs, but that was far from the truth. On January 9, 1998, we were married at a pastor's home with one of Michael's sister and her husband as witnesses.

We wanted to begin a family immediately and this proved to be an incredibly difficult and emotionally painful experience. In the States, I was already diagnosed with psoriasis and polycystic ovarian syndrome. I had no difficulty getting pregnant, but once I found out I was pregnant, I would miscarry within several days. The last time we attempted to get pregnant in South Africa, I miscarried on Mother's Day and was hospitalized for five days due to an infection. Michael and I were heartbroken.

Then in December 1999, we had an opportunity to move to Namibia. Michael was born in Namibia which was called South-West Africa back in 1968. Once Namibia became an independent country, everyone who was born in the former South-West Africa had dual citizenship. So in December, Michael received a call from his oldest sister who asked us to move to Namibia and we did. While Michael sorted out his paperwork (getting a copy of his "new" Namibian birth certificate, getting a Namibian passport, etc.), we lived at his sister's home. Despite the fact I didn't know Michael's sister, we hit it off immediately and I am eager to help her run her meat and fish shop that is attached to the back of her house. She is also aware of our previous problems having a baby and she encourages us to try again. Michael and I agree, but I tell him that if we miscarry again, I just can't try again.

Within a couple of months, we learn that I am pregnant and decide to keep the news a bit quiet. Sure enough within days of learning of the pregnancy, I begin to bleed. My doctor tells me to go to bed immediately and raise the bed up at the end with bricks. The bleeding stops quickly and several days later the doctor confirms that I am still pregnant. We are delighted and we begin to let more people know, including my parents, that I am pregnant. A couple of weeks later, Michael and I get our own flat and I find a new doctor in our new town. In my second trimester, I have some severe cramping and after a few hours in the hospital, I am released. In my third trimester, I am put on light rest.

When I am at 40 weeks, I have an exam because I have no hint that I'm going into labor. After the exam, I begin to bleed so I am referred to a hospital in Windhoek, the capital of Namibia. After an ultrasound and general exam, I am still bleeding so the decision is made to induce. Although I have horrible back labor pains, my cervix does not dilate. Several hours later, I am given a second dose with the same reaction. I then fall asleep and when I wake up, the right side of my abdomen is at least twice as larger as my left side. An emergency c-section is scheduled and as I am signing a bunch of forms and trying to talk to Michael at the same time, I am being prepped for surgery. Now my life and my unborn baby's life are in jeopardy. The sisters (nurses) ask me if there is only one opportunity to save me or the baby, whose life should be saved? With absolutely no hesitation, I tell them to save the baby. Michael absolutely freaks out, saying that we can have another baby. I can't speak for other expectant mothers, but to me my "role" as Mom is to sacrifice for my child. I have lived a life and it has been a wonderful life. I will not deprive my child to have a life to save mine. As I am wheeled into surgery, I accept the fact that I will die to save my child.

Since I was put under a general anesthetic, I can only tell you what I heard from the doctors and Michael afterwards. Because OUR situation was so dire, my incision was literally from hip to hip. When our son was born, he was dead. For some bizarre reason, Michael was asked to come into the surgical room while Jared was being revived and I was on the surgical table. Michael was brought in seeing blood dripping from my feet. I don't know how long my surgery lasted, but I do know that I either nearly died or died and was revived. Although I heard that I nearly bled out, I was also told that I didn't receive a blood transfusion. After the surgery was over, Michael was asked to visit me in recovery because I would not wake up. Someone asked him to say something that would grab my attention and all he could think of is tell me that we had a son. I know I heard it and yet it still took several more hours for me to fully wake up after being pumped full of drugs. I know I asked about our son and I spoke to my parents on our cell but I don't remember the conversation.

Our son was in the NICU because although the doctors confirmed that he was full-term, he only weighed four pounds. The theory was that at some point my placenta stopped feeding him. I was released from the hospital seven days later and our son remained for another two weeks. When our son was discharged, all the nurses and doctors who were there told us we were the "miracle" family. They honestly said that they never thought either one of us would leave the hospital alive.

Elizabeth looks at me and is clearly stunned. After thinking for a moment, Elizabeth tells me that she believes that this experience ended my life as I knew it and it opened my door of life with RSD. Now we are both stunned. How can an experience almost ten years ago have anything to do with my RSD?

Elizabeth explains that the reason why a near death or death experience can literally change a person's life is because of what it does to the hypothalamus. As defined in Wikipedia, "The hypothalamus (from Greek ὑπό = under and θάλαμος = room, chamber) is a portion of the brain that contains a number of small nuclei with a variety of functions. One of the most important functions of the hypothalamus is to link the nervous system to the endocrine

system via the pituitary gland (hypophysis).
The hypothalamus is located below the thalamus, just above
the brain stem. In the terminology of neuroanatomy, it
forms the ventral part of the diencephalon. All vertebrate
brains contain a hypothalamus. In humans, it is roughly the
size of an almond.

The hypothalamus is responsible for certain metabolic
processes and other activities of the Autonomic Nervous
System. It synthesizes and secretes neurohormones, often
called hypothalamic–releasing hormones, and these in turn
stimulate or inhibit the secretion of pituitary hormones. The
hypothalamus controls body temperature, hunger, thirst,
fatigue, and circadian cycles."

In layman's terms, Elizabeth explains that the hypothalamus
is the "computer" of the body. When someone has a near
death or death experience, the hypothalamus is
"reprogrammed" and, as a result, sometimes the person
experiences changes in healing, energy levels, body
temperature and metabolism. She asks me how I felt after I
had healed from my c–section and I admitted that I never
felt the same again. I began to gain weight, my energy level
was incredibly low and my sleeping patterns changed. I just
assumed that all of these changes were a direct result to
being a new Mom (and consequently having another child),
getting older, working, and moving around a lot. It never
occurred to me that the pain in my legs and exhaustion had
anything to do with an auto-immune disease. Elizabeth
says she honestly believes that RSD slowly developed in my
body over time, masking itself as other ailments as it
normally does. However when I had my accident in July, it
was so dramatic that my symptoms increased dramatically
and the diagnosis was finally made.

So how have I coped with this information? Very well.
Honestly, there were only two options available on that
fateful day for me on 12-12-00....I could die and remain
dead or I could live and have RSD. I choose life with RSD. I
have far too much to live for and so many blessings in my
life. I will be the first to admit that when I was first

diagnosed, my depression was terrible. It was like I was in a pit and I simply could not get out of my own way to climb out of it. But slowly with the help of a couple of fabulous friends, my husband, Elizabeth, my family and a lot of soul-searching, I climbed out of it. I know that I will never be back in that pit but it was part of my grieving process that I just had to go through back then. Absolutely the one question that has stunned me over and over again is "Do I blame Jared for my RSD?" What??????? How in the world would I EVER blame my first born for my RSD?????? My child, my baby, did not cause my RSD. Frankly, I don't blame anyone for my RSD. It just HAPPENED. Without fail, this question has ALWAYS been asked by a mother. The first time it happened, I was so stunned that I could barely speak. Now when I am asked this question, I have to put my hands behind my back so that only my mouth does the lashing. Frankly, it gives me great comfort that I share my RSD anniversary with Jared's birthday because it is always a celebration. It is a celebration of living......of both of us being miracles, of being survivors. Together, we made it out alive out of that hospital and since then I have given birth to another miracle child and our family lives here in the States. I have a fabulous RSD doctor and have made lots of RSD friends online on Facebook. I am thrilled to celebrate my twelve years of RSD on 12-12-12 as our son Jared turns 12 years old. I wouldn't want it any other way.

HOW CRPS AFFECTS THE FAMILY
STORIES OF CAREGIVERS

Barb's Story:
My beautiful daughter Stacey was diagnosed with RSD/CRPS in September of 2009. She was cleaning the bottom of her oak kitchen table,where there was dog and cat hair on one of the kegs.The table slipped and landed on the top of her right foot. She went to ER where she was told there was no break and the doctor put her in a boot and on crutches. She was in burning pain right away. We saw the family doctor in 3 days and because she had drop foot already he decided to cast her. The cast was on for 6 weeks. During this time Stacey was in horrible pain. We just didn't know what was going on. The doctor took the cast off and she had horrible discoloration and her foot was so swollen.My daughter worked full-time as a certified nursing assistant,working the night shift so she could still be home with her kids. She was very active in their school as well as after school activities .She took care of her home and loved gardening,and playing with her kids. She loves animals and she has 3 of them.

Stacey was a very active young girl as well.She was in cheerleading gymnastics, Girl Scouts as well as field hockey. Her whole life changed that year in 2009 as well as ours. My daughter was sent to an orthopedic doctor who sent her to physical therapy, where she was put through horrible,very painful exercises. Additionally they were icing her foot. Meanwhile her foot was blue and purple and swollen and very painful. From there she was sent to pain management doctor who told us "you have RSD."

What is RSD? We never heard of that. He explained to us what it was but we I look back now were in shock as he spoke. He decided to do blocks in her spine. She had 10 of those.The relief only lasted for a few hours. She was started on narcotics ,which was then I realized I had lost the daughter I used to know. Her whole personality changed.

The RSD was spreading to her other foot and leg .Block after block,medication after medication she continued to get worse. My grandchildren could not understand what was happening to their Mommy. The pain management doctor did an epidural of lidocaine. I took care of her at home with that. She was numb below the waist but still able to function (a walking epidural). Unfortunately she could only have that in for 5 days. She got so much relief from that, The day I was supposed to take her back to the pain management doctor, she wouldn't even go because the pain was so much gone. I talked to the pain management doctor. He was a wonderful doctor. He agreed to let her have it one more day. It was suggested she have a spinal column stimulator implanted. Stacey was very unsure of this and her husband wanted her to have this procedure done as soon as possible as he thought she would be cured. She agreed to it. It was the worst thing she could have done. Her RSD started spreading all over and the site of the stimulator was burning so badly. She had it removed She saw Dr S in 2010 and WOW were our eyes opened to what RSD really is. By now my beautiful Stacey was wheelchair bound she could not walk. She was loaded up with medications that were not working.

Dr S. Suggested Ketamine.. As for me ,her Mom, well I can't say how helpless i was felling. A Mom is supposed to be able to help her children and make them better. I thought I was going to lose it. But then I looked at her very scared face and the look on my grandkids faces and i knew I had to be strong and do whatever it took to make sure she received the best of care. Stacey is our youngest and from the time she was 18 she has been suffering. .She lost her first born son, our Bandon, who was born with a heart defect. She watched her baby suffer through surgeries after surgery. We lived at the hospital for most of the 13 months we had our little Angel. And as Stacey's mom I could not take that pain away from her as I so much wanted to.

Now she had 2 healthy children and her life was doing great when POUNCE that table changed everything. As her mom I cry daily but not that she can see. I search and I search for ways to get her through the days. This RSD has changed all of us as a family .We worry about her. We worry about our grandkids, as this is so very hard for them. They cry in their sleep and don't even realize it. I have heard them on many of times and it breaks my heart. Seeing your active, fun loving, smiling, beautiful daughter, gone is heart breaking. That is how it feels; like she is gone. The pain is on her face, the the smile is gone, her body isn't hers anymore. I think if I'm feeling like this way, much pain are my grandkids feeling?????

There are times when I look at my beautiful daughter and I ask GOD why why can you please give this disease to me,PLEASE! I beg all the time. Watching my Brandon suffer. Seeing my Stacey as his Mom who could do nothing to save him. The pain of all that and now once again she is suffering. I am watching her and feeling of so helpless. This is just not fair. I want to take it all away and give my grandkids their Mommy back.I try so hard to keep the children upbeat and hopeful that their mommy will one day be better and be able to walk again. Soon she will do the things with them as she used to do. They miss her and she misses them badly.

I took Kylie (my granddaughter) shopping this weekend because she needed some things. I looked in my daughter's eyes and saw the hurt and the sadness because she wanted to be the one to take her. Right now she is in so much pain that she can barely get out of bed. I saw the sadness in Kylie's eyes as well. his is heartbreaking for a mom and mom mom. All the dreams I had for my daughter have been all taken away, All of them. Now all I want to do is fix her. I want to make her better take this on myself. I have lived my life but she hasn't. As I lay awake night after night thinking and seeing my Stacey as a child; her great big beautiful smile is so very vivid in my brain iI see her walking, running, happy, and smiling. I see how happy she was when her children were born. I see her running and jumping with them,smiling all the time. I see her as she was when we were on vacation as a child. I see all the fun times and see her smiling.I want it back. I can't make it happen. I want my grandkids to smile like they used to do as well. They have learned to be so independent and so very helpful and compassionate, loving and kind. For these things I'am so very grateful, but not for the way they learned this RSD takes so much away from the patient and so much away from the family. I never thought my beautiful Stacey would have to suffer like this.

I look back at the day she was born and how happy we were to have a daughter. I would hold her and cuddle her and rock her and sing to her as her Mom I I never,ever thought that my precious baby girl would suffer as she has. Losing her baby my goodness isn't that pain enough. Now just when her life was going so well ZAP it is gone. She now spends her days in excruciating pain, lying in bed wishing she would be better even ever so slightly Mostly she would want to be walking so she could be with her children, take them shopping and drive them where they want to be. She misses playing ball with Zach and football with him. She is missing out on dancing with Kylie as she so much lives to do. I pray always for a cure always.

Nicole's Story; How RSD Changed our life
How has RSD changed this family? RSD entered into our home in the darkness of night. Nicole was 15 years old – a competitive dance, basketball player, alter server, involved at home, neighborhood, school and community. She is the girl next door with a killer smile always. Nicole was a sophomore in high school in an accelerated program called Classical Academy and she received all A's – a remarkable young lady. As I started out saying, RSD crept in at night while she was asleep. Nicole woke with a stiff neck and another of her infamous sinus infections. Off to the doctor she went. This time was different though. The pain and stiffness spread down her back. She lost the ability read; lights, sounds, smells and motions were all troublesome to her. She was told she needed to leave school as she was not well enough to attend. Nicole did everything that was asked of her from medications to physical therapy to psychologist to a multitude of doctors and any and all tests

requested. I researched and researched and made call after to call trying to find out why a seemingly healthy young lady is stopped dead in her tracks and how do I help her get her life back and quickly.

Nicole had been seen by the best and the brightest some would report and for two and a half years she was told things would be better in 3 to 5 years. As the third year was approaching, she was getting worse and worse and the pain had spread to her left leg and left arm. Her body was doing very odd things like her left arm jerked while I was driving her to appointments that would smash me in the chest and knock the wind out of me and she sat stunned and in tremendous pain. Some of these brilliant doctors wanted her to further isolate and move to the back of the car. I kept asking, why not stop them. Aren't there medications that can prevent this from happening. Repeatedly being told that the risks outweighed the benefits. The risk that no one took into consideration was the ability to use her left arm and the kicker – she was a lefty. She has converted to being a righty as she had no other options. Doctors quickly say she wasn't a true lefty then as she was able to change hands. I would love to see someone change from lefty to righty as Nicole did while learning geometry. I will say it again – she is remarkable. Nicole now uses a power wheelchair as she has no stamina or endurance for all that her body has endured. I am so happy to say she has left this fall to be a freshman at Providence College (PC). She is doing very well and thriving. Providence College has been instrumental in giving her her life back. When we drove on to campus for her very first meeting with the disability coordinator, she announced in the driveway –"I love it here. This is where I want to go." Many other meetings took place and while suffering from a spinal leak and laying flat in the living room on an air mattress, this courageous young woman wrote her essays and submitted her college applications. By the way she was accepted to all six school she applied, but PC is the only one that has her heart. How has RSD affected our family?

Our family was changed forever 12/20/2001 when Nicole's dad died of colon cancer after 66 days of being ill. A 40 year old man, who just found the house of his dreams, had the job he had been working towards, the truck he always desired, a wife and two beautiful daughters. The girls and I trudged on and managed sadly without him. Nicole wanted more of her own money and started as a mother's helper in the neighborhood when she was 10 years old. She loved Aeropostle clothing and wanted an iPod and Nicole found a way to make that happen. This mother's helper position turned into a very good paying position for two families with special needs children and she was a patient care attendant. Her older sister, Caitlin, loved school, being in plays and being a teenager. As Nicole got sick, Cait and Nicole went from being sisters who got along very well, to girls who couldn't stand to be in the same room. Cait looks at Nicole's illness with deep seeded fear and also has resentment as from a teenagers perspective I am giving more to her younger sibling than I am to Cait. The effect was so profound on Cait, that just two months prior to Cait's High School graduation, Cait moved out in protest to how RSD had taken over our lives. I am happy to say she recently returned home. Cait being 20, makes 20 years old assumptions and mistakes. This is definitely a work in progress. Nicole and Cait do not enjoy the closeness they once did. RSD is partly to blame. I hope as they mature and move on with life they find the closeness they once shared. As a mother, I unfortunately don't have much say to their relationship.

When the girls' Dad died, I was a stay at home mom as he was a latchkey kid and he refused to have his girls brought up that way. I loved being home with the girls and was a part of their school activities, church activities and extra activities. I am fortunate that I was able to continue for the most part after his death, but I returned to school while they were in school. I am one of those people still that doesn't know what they want to be when they grow up. I started taking classes to be a teacher as with the girls being 8 and 9 years old, the schedule would be grand. I then changed to being an interpreter for American Sign Language. The time commitments of an interpreter were exceedingly more difficult than I had anticipates. I changed finally to Radiology Technology and finally graduated in May, 2009. Unfortunately Nicole was so ill at the time, that looking for employment was out of the question. I took my test and passed my boards and I was a certified licensed technologist in the Commonwealth of Massachusetts. Nicole illness progressed. Doctor appointments, Physical therapy, Occupational Therapy and anything else I could find to try to help my daughter was our life from May 2009 until January 30, 2012. Now on January 30, I didn't stop my pursuit, instead an angel entered our world and the madness began to end. WE found a pain specialist in Rhode Island and he has been instrumental to ending the madness. This is not to say that Nicole s cured or Nicole lives a "normal" life of a 19 year old. The madness that enters with RSD. It's all in your head. You will be better in 3 to 5 years. You just have to this or that. We met a wonderful doctor who told Nicole that RSD is real and not in her head. It is making your autonomic system go out of kilter, and best of all. He had options, he had a belief in her and what she was going through. As a parent that had been fighting a multitude of doctors in very prestigious establishments, I was and still am so grateful for this precious man to have entered our life. When he saw her veins and how bad they are, he ordered a port-a-cath to be placed and ordered no more needle sticks from now own. Nicole had been having 18 to 20 convulsive episodes daily that were kept at bay with fluids and he made that happen. Nicole hasn't had a convulsive episode since May. She hasn't fainted since the beginning of June. He started her on new medications and they worked. In fact, they worked so well that I no longer had to give her air hugs I could actually place my arms gently around my baby and I can kiss her cheek.

This wonderful doctor had another doctor her wanted her to see for the autonomic issues and this doctor is also a dream. He started her on medication that has stopped a lot of her issues with her autonomic system. Her last appointment he even asked Nicole if she would be in touch with other patients like her as she is "the poster child" for

POTS. Next Nicole went to the physical therapist that this wonderful doctor uses. Physical therapy that had results is what Nicole is finally getting. For me, I am thrilled to see doctors working together and seeing a patient before them and dealing with whatever symptoms her body decides to have. I get to breath now. I no longer have shoulders for earring. I am relaxing.

Since I didn't work after getting my Radiology Technology license, getting a job 3 years later wasn't going to happen, especially in this economic climate we are in currently. I was able to go back to school online and I am in the process of becoming a CT Scan Technologist and I will hopefully be working soon after I am tested and licensed.

RSD has taken a lot away from Nicole's life, but it has taught us all just how truly strong we are, to believe in ourselves even if no one else is – and that even counts if the other person has a whole lot of letters after their name, doctors can be incorrect. RSD is a double edge sword. I will never say I am glad it entered our world, but since it is here and has taken up residence for how ever long, RSD will not be in charge. Nicole is in charge and she is in Rhode Island living life again. I am learning to live with her an hour and a half away and not needing as so much as she once did. Her sister is at home with me. Every day we get up and try to make it the best day possible – just like most every other person alive.

Our Daughter Jessica's Battle with RSD
By Janice and Lee

When Nancy Cotterman asked me to contribute to her novel in May of 2012, I was unable to write due to what our daughter's RSD had done to my emotional state. The privilege of meeting Nancy was the beginning of our salvation. Our daughter, Jessica (Jess) had a failed bunionectomy in May 2005. The podiatrist said it might take up to a year until she was totally healed. Her pain level seemed to be out of the norm. When she asked him for a refill on her pain medicine, which was Vicodin ES, he gave it to her but he said that he had never performed a bunionectomy and had a patient ask for a refill on their pain medication. After a period of time, he began giving her cortisone shots in her toe. Jess said they were extremely painful. This went on for numerous months until he suggested the reason for her pain was that the toe next to her big toe was too long and he wanted to cut off the last joint in her second toe. Her father quickly took her out of the office and never went back. Jessica had no movement in her left big toe so we felt the next step was to see an orthopedic surgeon. At this point, she had undiagnosed RSD. She had major swelling on the lateral and underside of her left foot. We all know the last thing you want to do when you have RSD is have surgery. Why did it not ever enter these doctors minds? Next, the orthopedic surgeon operated on her big toe.This occurred in August 2006. He removed scar tissue and she did regain most movement. Along with the movement came major discoloration from blue to purple to red. After this surgery is when the pain and RSD symptoms skyrocketed. The pain was now from her toe to her groin. She had marked sensitivity to touch, vibrations, and allodynia. This is when our journey to hell and back began.

At this time, I, her mother, was being treated by a pain doctor/anesthesiologist receiving spinal injections to attempt to avoid a second back operation, a laminectomy. My husband and I figured that would be a good doctor to take her to see. She was diagnosed with RSD in five minutes. We were ecstatic, a diagnosis, a reason for her pain. Little did we know what we were in store for. We came straight home and looked up RSD on the computer and were in shock. It is now January 2007, 20 months after her bunion surgery. The anesthesiologist sent her for x-rays, an MRI, a triple phase bone scan and nerve conduction tests to confirm her diagnosis of RSD. Unfortunately, her diagnosis was accurate. Jessica began a series of fluoroscopic guided sympathetic nerve blocks. All they did was hurt her back with no improvement whatsoever. She continued these until April. All the anesthesiologist wanted to do was cut her pain medicine down.

I then took her to see a neurologist who of course confirmed the diagnosis, but informed us that he does not treat RSD. He stated that it was too complicated. He told us that the leading doctor to treat RSD was Dr Robert Schwartzman who was located in Philadelphia, but it would take two years to get an appointment. Upon chatting, we learned that my husbands uncle, a retired neurologist in Philadelphia knew Dr Schwartzman and would be able to get us an appointment much sooner. As soon as we got in the car, we called him. He called us back later that day and informed us that we had an appointment in two weeks. It is now April of 2007. Dr Schwartzman examined Jessica, confirmed RSD and wanted her to have a special MRI at the Hospital for Special Surgery in New York City. He felt there was a possibility that she had a neuroma that was maintaining her RSD. In May, we packed up and headed to NYC. The MRI showed that she had avascular necrosis, which is a lack of blood supply going to her toe. They said this can be very serious and recommended a hip to toe bone marrow transplant. We saw Dr Daniel Richman, a renowned pain management specialist as well as a tremendous foot and ankle specialist, Dr Andrew Elliott. He performed two different kinds of tests on Jess the next day and agreed with the opinion of Dr. Richman. We didn't plan on staying overnight, so we had no clothes with us. We slept in our clothes, bought toothbrushes and toothpaste. We had to change our flight home and even though it was for medical reasons, they charged us $500 to change our flights. We were irate, but what could we do? She finished her junior year of college in May and was forced to drop out with a GPA of 3.99. This broke our hearts. Our advise to others is that when you have pain that is out of the norm, go straight to your primary care physician for a referral to an anesthesiologist. Her primary care physician changed her medication from Vicodin ES to Percocet 10/325. After a period of time, he put her on a fentanyl patch as well as valium, cymbalta and 2400 mg of neurontin daily. Of course, she didn't start with that high level. The neurontin was eventually changed to lyrica. Our cleaning lady recommended us to see a new pain doctor where her daughter was being treated. We liked him very much. He seemed to be warm, compassionate and quite knowledgeable about RSD.

In July 2007, Jess had her surgery at the Hospital for Special Surgeries by Dr. Andrew Elliott. She was in the ICU for 5 days. In addition to the bone marrow transplant, he performed a cryoneurolisis, which is a freezing of the nerve and also buried that nerve in the bone. Additionally, he was able to get the pin out of her toe that the podiatrist inserted and the orthopedic surgeon in Pittsburgh, where we live, was unable to get out. She was on ketamine the entire time in the hospital. We don't know the dosage, but upon returning home her RSD seemed to be gone away for one month. She was only in post-surgical pain. Slowly but surely all the RSD symptoms returned and the nightmare continued once again.

After healing from her surgery, her pain doctor in Pittsburgh suggested that she enroll in a 6 week rehabilitation program that took place 3 times a week for 6 hours each day. Jess did as he recommended and received physical therapy, occupational therapy and psychological services.It is now 2008. She had been receiving private physical therapy since 2005 when she felt able to get out of bed. She returned home with extreme exhaustion and crawled into bed after every day she attended this program. At this point, she needed to be driven everywhere she went. She hated to ride in the car due to the vibrations. She missed so many family functions and holidays because of the extreme pain she would endure after a car ride. She missed Thanksgiving, family birthdays and Jewish Holiday dinners, to name a few. Of course, we always brought her food home. When she completed the program, she felt sicker than when it began. She spent most of her time in bed from 2007 through 2009. Our beautiful daughter was sleeping her life away. At this point, all of her friends deserted her except her best friend who was like a sister to her. Unfortunately, she took a special education position in Hawaii upon graduating college. Talking on the phone isn't quite the same, although she always came to see Jess numerous times when she visited Pittsburgh twice a year. She is like a second daughter to us. Her other so-called friends didn't understand her illness and never attempted to do so. They had all turned 21 and their interest was drinking, bar-hopping and getting drunk. This wouldn't interest Jessica even if she was well. We lived with a very sick and lonely daughter who spent a lot of time crying, constantly asking why me? Why me? As her parents we asked the same question, why her? We had now lost faith in religion.

Jessica has a brother Michael, who is 3 years younger than her. They used to be very close. Once Jess had RSD their relationship deteriorated drastically. Mike was definitely embarrassed of her as she had gained a good 50 pounds. Lee and I felt like our close family was being torn apart and we were deeply hurt. Jessica was beautiful from the day she was born, with the most beautiful long eyelashes we had ever seen on a newborn, never funny looking at all. When she was a teenager she was built like a brick house, as the saying goes. She never once visited him at college nor did he invite her or encourage her to do so. He went to Robert Morris University, which is located 30 minutes from our house. Mike lived there and only came home on Thanksgiving, Christmas Break, Spring Break, Easter Break and summers.(and an occasional good home-cooked meal) My children only got along when they did not live under the same roof. Michael wasn't very interested in learning about RSD and felt that taking care of Jessica took our time away from him. Fortunately, he has always been an independent child but Jess' father, Lee, and I, her mother, Janice did not feel that Michael was deserted in any way. We were saddened by the fact that our wonderful, close-knit family was being torn apart. To this day, I am not sure he ever even read an article to understand and learn about RSD. He constantly called her names. We believe lazy was the biggest one and told her that she never tried to do anything to help herself. At this point, he was too young and immature and showed Jess no compassion whatsoever. Jess' dad had developed severe depression and anxiety. Mike blamed Jess for this. In March of 2008, Lee had a nervous breakdown. He felt he needed to get away, so he went to visit his brother and sister-in-law in Chicago. When the day came to leave, he didn't want to go, but I encouraged him to do so and told him he will feel better when he gets there. He left on a Friday and was supposed to return on Monday. He called me when he arrived and he sounded ok, not great, but ok. When he called me Saturday night, it was a totally different scenario. He sounded terrible. They had gone out to dinner and had to leave the restaurant because Lee felt so terrible. I told him to take a valium and go to sleep. He wanted to come home. I encouraged him to try and make it through the weekend and told him we will see how you feel tomorrow. Sunday, around noon, I was out to brunch with my son, Mike. Lee called crying so hysterically that I couldn't understand a word he was saying. I asked him to please put his brother on the phone. His brother said he wants to come home but we can take care of him here. I know my husband. We had been married almost 23 years at this point. I told his brother to get him on a plane ASAP. He kept arguing with me that he's his brother. He's known him his entire life. We can can take care of him. I was adamant and of course he got him right on a plane. His brother resented both of us, but especially me, for quite some time after my forcefulness to get Lee home. He definitely didn't understand anxiety and depression. Once Lee got on the plane, he felt better. As soon as he saw me, he thanked me over and over for my persistence. He knew that I would know what was best for him. He was unable to work on Monday and by Tuesday morning he was a mess to put it bluntly. I still remember calling his sister at 6:08 AM for help. Not only does she have her MSW, but she has had her own private practice and numerous psychologists and psychiatrists. She got him an emergency appointment with a psychiatrist that very day! Of course, I took him. He was unable to drive anyway. After that he spent many months in therapy from a psychiatrist and psychologist who confirmed his diagnosis of SEVERE anxiety and depression. He has worked hard to be as healthy as he can be. Lee is a dentist, a professional man, and he blamed himself for Jessica's RSD. How could he let her have bunion surgery. He should have not allowed it. He expressed this over and over and over again. I always told him it was not his fault. I never felt I was to blame for her illness. She was 19, hated the way her foot looked, shoes started hurting her and her foot was painful. There is only so much control you can have over a 19-year-old's decisions. I felt it was her genetic make-up and if she didn't get RSD from her bunion surgery, she would have gotten it a different way, from a fall, a paper cut, some way, some how.

I reacted in a totally different manner, although both of us were broken-hearted. There is nothing worse that watching your child suffer, cry uncontrollably, writhe in pain with all the horrific symptoms of RSD. The only thing worse is having your child die. Something that Jess mentioned from time to time, but she never meant it. We were never worried about suicide. It was just an expression. Lee and I were social drinkers. Before Jessica had RSD, we would have a few cocktails after work a couple nights a week and once on the weekend. I was the manager at his dental office for over 20 years. I had my second laminectomy by a different surgeon in November of 2006. This surgeon said it was the worst herniated disc he ever operated on. I had undiagnosed scoliosis from childhood which definitely compromised my condition as well as degenerative disc disease and arthritis. I never got out of pain, but I never stopped working. I hobbled around and it took my mind off my pain. I began drinking every night to numb my physical pain and my emotional pain. This went on for 4 years. I took care of Jess during the day on my days off and missed many days of work because I couldn't bare to leave her. Working for my husband, I definitely had job security. I took her to every doctor appointment in Pittsburgh, Philadelphia and New York. Of course Lee also came for her surgery. We took shifts at the hospital. I always had the early shift, first of all because I am up early and secondly I had to be home by 4 o'clock to begin my drinking. Lee and Jess never gave me a hard time about my drinking. My son was a different story. He hated my drinking, but was at college most of the time. Therefore he didn't have to face it every day. Maybe another reason why he never came home much. We always talked, texted every day. We had always been a close family. It's not always the best thing to be parents and friends with your children, but that's how we were. It just came naturally. Although we must admit we were sometimes told things by them that we didn't want to know. It's called TMI, too much information. Michael moved home from college in May of 2011. That was an adjustment for everyone. It was hard for Jess as he picked on her constantly. I continued my drinking. I would fall asleep on my deck, burn holes in my clothes as I smoke, fall off my chair and fell asleep in my plate. I had two strong drinks but I was taking percocet and valium daily for my severe back. It was not a good mix. Michael used to tell me it was like I had a split personality. It was like I was a different person during the day than I was at night. I couldn't wait until 4 or 5 o'clock came every day. I counted the hours but I never drank during the day. Then the shit hit the fan. Mike gave me an ultimatum and told me that if I continue to drink that when he has children one day, they will not be allowed to have anything to do with me. I was always there for Jessica during the day, but after Lee worked all day, he would come home to a drunk wife and had to totally take over. He held her night after night after night and would hold her foot for her because it was so cold.

Family is one of the most important things in my life. I am lucky to have both of my parents still living and I have a sister who is my best friend in addition to my husband and children. I told Mike that I couldn't quit cold turkey. I was afraid I would get sick, go into withdrawal, something would happen to me. I promised him I would quit drinking, but please let me do it my own way. Starting in the middle of May, I cut down my drinking to once a week and had my last drink on August 11, 2011, 4 days before I was scheduled to have a 4-level lumbar fusion due to multiple pinched nerves and bulging discs. I am proud to say I am 13 months sober and loving it. I don't want to be that person anymore so it's very easy not to drink. I never even think about it. I will always be forever grateful to my wonderful son who saved my life. I am part of the family again, being together and remembering conversations, good times, bad times. Many thanks Michael.

To back track a little bit, I reconnected with one of my best friends from college in 2008. We had been in touch on the computer occasionally for about 10 to 15 years, but hadn't seen him since I graduated college in 1980. For my 50th birthday, I went to visit him in Sarasota, FL. with my college roommate in February. It was like I saw him yesterday and the first night I was there, we stayed up to 3 o'clock in the morning talking. We talked on the phone often that year. The year of 2009 was my year of running away and escaping because of Jessica's devastating illness. I went to Sarasota 5 times that year. I have the most wonderful, understanding husband in the world who understood my need to get away. He was quite different from me. He could never leave Jessica. That is what was the icing on the cake to cause his nervous breakdown. He discovered that he could not leave her. We rarely went out as we would never have a good time because we were constantly worrying about her. We still always tried to go out to dinner for family birthdays, but stopped socializing with our friends. We definitely lost friends due to the fact that we just couldn't go out anymore and leave her. We may have gone out a few times a year. There were 2 weddings we didn't go to. We responded yes, but when the day came we cancelled or no-showed.

When I visited my friend in Sarasota, we had lots of good times. We reconnected instantly and it was like no time had passed since we had seen each other. Unfortunately he got to see the worst side of me. He saw me fall, drop and break a wine glass, fall asleep at dinner and the worst night of all. We were out to dinner and I couldn't finish my dinner. I rarely did. I thought there was a take out box on the table and took my plate and dumped it on the table. After a few visits, he realized I needed help and left me letters explaining my behavior, telling me I needed help and left me the phone number of Alcoholics Anonymous. When I left the last time, I knew I was no longer welcome to visit him. Approximately 2-4 weeks after my lumbar fusion, he wrote me a letter saying I hope you get better from your surgery Janice, but do not call me, text me or e-mail me. Get help and get better. I was devastated beyond belief. Family and friends are so important to me. He was like the big brother I never had and I felt like he had deserted me. I had already stopped drinking but a few weeks or a month meant nothing to him.He told me to call him in a year. I never stopped calling or e-mailing him, but he never responded. I cried my eyes out every day, hysterical beyond belief. We had been friends for 30 years. This was really tough love. In the end, my good friend Marty played a major role in keeping me sober. A special thank you to Marty for helping me to stay sober. I guess I am one of the rare people who never went to AA or had therapy of any kind. All I needed was tough love from those who loved me enough to give it to me. Marty and I are great friends again and keep in touch on a regular basis.

Sometime in late 2009 or early 2010, Jessica finally received her disability which allowed her to receive medicare benefits. It took a year and a half. Due to my numerous back surgeries, I am also on disability. I can't sit for long periods of time and can't stand for more than 5 minutes or so. I can walk better than I can stand. I haven't been able to cook my family dinner in over a year. Cooking was one of my greatest passions in life. I felt and still somewhat trapped in my own body. Recently, I am able to cook a side dish. My surgeon gave me a year and a half to 2 year recovery as I fell asleep driving on New Years Day and have fallen numerous times. I received my disability in 4 months and it tok Jess a year and a half. There is something very wrong with our health system. They do not realize or understand the debilitation and devastation to one's life that RSD causes.

In 2009, we finally were able to get Jess out of bed. I was becoming too sick to work and we felt if she worked voluntarily at her dad's dental office, it would give her a purpose in life and distract her from her severe burning, throbbing, aching pain. She took over my job and began running the reception area of the office along with her aunt. The plan worked. She loved it! She started working 2 hours a day, then 4 and now works 6 or 7 hours a day. At the beginning, she was so physically and mentally exhausted that she would come home and sleep for hours. At this point, she was on a lot of medication. Her pain doctor had just disappeared one day and we were desperate to find a new one. The new doctor didn't know what to do for her. She had been on morphine from the last pain doctor and the new doctor just kept increasing it to the point where she was taking 500 mg of morphine per day.He surely didn't have the compassion or bedside manner of her last pain doctor, but we couldn't afford to be particular. Some pain doctors just perform procedures and don't write narcotics at all.

2010 was the year that Jess discovered the RSD/CRPS Ketamine Club on Facebook. We both joined. It was very helpful emotionally. Jessica found people to relate to and so did I. This is where we met the wonderful, amazing Nancy Cotterman and many other compassionate people. They are too numerous to mention. A special thanks to all the administrators, people with RSD and their families who were willing to share their stories.

In April of 2012, a light bulb went off in my head out of nowhere. I remembered from being at Dr. Schwartzman's office back in 2007 that ketamine infusions are covered by medicare. I screamed with excitement to Jessica and she remembered too. We were elated as the cost was $50,000 in 2007 and not covered by our Blue Cross/Blue Shield insurance. We were not aware of being persistent and appealing to the insurance company back then. I immediately called Lee's uncle and he got us an appointment with one of Dr. Schwartzman's associates in 4 days. It sure is helpful to have connections. We never had an appointment with Dr. Tabby, Dr. Schwartzman's associate that day. Jessica was already scheduled to begin her pre-ketamine testing which consisted of neuro-psychological tests and cardiac work-up. That day she had her psychological testing. We discovered that she had a memory loss and had many family members who have some form of ambidextrousness. These signs are consistent with people who have RSD. We had to make another trip to Philadelphia for her cardiac work-up and scheduled it as soon as we got home. Jessica was not happy to have a port inserted and be hospitalized for her ketamine infusion, but she was at the point where she would do anything possible to be fortunate enough to have a ketamine infusion. This is when Nancy interjected and told Jessica there is a great doctor in Miami, Florida, Dr. Dennis Patin, who does ketamine infusions on an out-patient basis and does not insert a port. We must thank you Nancy for guiding us in the right direction, being patient with Jessica, and putting up with her endless phone calls and texts. I quickly called his office and we were able to get an appointment in 2-3 weeks. This was May 2012. Coincidentally, Nancy was in Miami accompanying a friend who was having a ketamine infusion when Jessica had her initial appointment with Dr. Patin and we got to meet her. Jess was elated. We scheduled her ketamine infusion for the week of July 30, 2012. By this time, we had discovered Mercy Medical Airlift who flies patients receiving medical treatments to other cities who cannot afford it. They find a sponsor to pay for their flight. We had depleted all of our savings over the years due to Jessica's medical treatments, prescriptions, numerous airplane trips, hotels and had a terrible accountant. We lost our house in 2011, two and a half years before it was paid off. We had a beautiful 4 bedroom, two and a half bathroom home with a family room and a park-like yard. Obviously, we have changed accountants and now rent a house. But as we all know, home is where your family lives. It's not a bad house, but the houses are close together, the bedrooms are smaller and the yard is one quarter of our old home.

July 30th finally arrived. Lee, Jessica and I had flown in the day before as Jessica needed to be at the hospital at 7:30. The hotel was only two blocks away from the Sylvester Comprehensive Cancer Center, where Dr. Patin is located. It is very convenient as they have a shuttle that runs every half hour starting early in the morning until noon and then resumes again around 4 o'clock. The first day of treatment is only half dose to make sure the patient doesn't have a bad reaction to ketamine. Jessica was also given versed, ativan and zophran to control the side effects of ketamine, which are nausea, anxiety and possibly hallucinations. She came home from her first day of treatment 100% RSD free. We couldn't believe our eyes and ears. Jess was tired. That's it. After the third day of treatment, she didn't want to back. She wanted to go to the beach, but she knew she couldn't. She finished her five days of treatment. Dr. Patin informed her that he has never had a patient become RSD pain-free after one day of treatment. He said that he doesn't have a crystal ball, but he believes Jessica may fall into that rare category of never needing a ketamine treatment again. Since that time, he has changed his mind and wants her to just have one assurance booster. Jessica is in 100% remission. Her toe hurts from arthritis and her leg aches from not using it for so long. She walks our German Shepherd very large 9 month old puppy a mile every day. She unloads the dishwasher, helps bring in the groceries and put them away and helps with dinner. As bad as RSD is, Jess was lucky that hers never spread past her toe to her groin, while so many people suffer from full body RSD.

We feel a miracle has occurred. Our beautiful daughter, who missed so many years of her teenage-young adult years has her life back. She has lost so much weight that she is half the size of her former self. She is going back to college in January to finish her undergraduate degree and then continue on to get her MSW, Masters in Social Work. She receives great pleasure from helping others, she always has, so this is a field that is appropriate for her. Our beautiful daughter will have a husband and family one day. I, personally had forgotten what a special, unique person she is. It got lost and trapped in her pain. She is the kindest, most compassionate, loving person we have ever met. We are not saying this because she is our daughter. She has always been this way. From the time she was a toddler, she told me every day of my life how much she loves me and I am the best mother in the world. She did this until she was about 15 or 16 and then I became the best mother in the world and outer space. How many children express that special kind of love? How many parents can say that about their child? She is 26 now and no longer says it every day, but we know the feelings are there. She is equally as close to her father. Jessica and Michael are close once again and have that special bond that brothers and sisters share.

A special thank you must be included to my sister, her Aunt Susie who is like her second mother. She constantly offered her time, love and devotion. As she doesn't sleep well due to fibromyalgia, she talked to Jessica for hours in the middle of the night when Jess was writhing in pain. Talking to my sister calmed Jessica down and surely made her feel loved. This continued for a period of 2–3 years. My sister always was there for Jessica when we needed a break or just couldn't handle the stress that RSD causes.

We are realistic that her RSD could come back, but we don't dwell on it. If it does return, we are told it will NEVER be as bad as it was prior to her receiving ketamine. She will get another ketamine infusion or booster. With the way she responds to ketamine, her RSD would go into remission again. This is what we have been told by professionals.

This is the miracle story of Jessica HOPE Feinberg and her devastating battle with RSD. What an appropriate name. Our greatest wish is that her story will give hope to others who suffer from RSD.

(From Nancy: as of 12/31/13 Jessica Hope remains in remission)

Sue
Westerville, Ohio
This is my story of how RSD has affected our lives.

May 30th, 2008, not only changed Katie's life forever but changed my life and that of the rest of her family as well. Katie suffered a severe foot injury that was bad enough in and of itself, but the resulting RSD is a kind of 'hell' that none of us could have anticipated. Her fractures healed but RSD prevailed. She is an RN as am I. She was supposed to be off that May 30th but volunteered to trade days with a coworker so that he could take his family camping. I have wished so many times that this one moment in time could be undone. How different all of our lives, especially Katie's, would have been. That is not possible of course and all any of us can do is deal with RSD the best we can and move forward. But as her Mom, I so wish I could fix things for her. That is what moms do. They are supposed to fix things.

I have had too many conversations to count with Katie over the past few years since her injury. I am her Mom, her advisor, her "therapist", her driver, her caretaker when needed, and her shoulder to lean on and to cry on. We have cried together and gathered strength from each other. I am so proud of Katie. She has had to deal with not only the injury but all of the issues of RSD. The pain, burning, sleep deprivation, anger and frustration over just having to continue to deal with everything is sometimes too much for even the very strongest person. The uncertainties of what may be ahead is probably the thing that is most scary. The ebb and flow of her multiple symptoms effect her day to day and sometimes change hour to hour. RSD becomes all consuming. It effects everything and multiple parts of your body. It is difficult to explain to others when from the outside Katie appears so normal.

There isn't a day or night that goes by without thoughts about Katie. My prayers have been endless that she will have a good night or that she gets through her day at work and then that the evening/night after a day at work is OK. I wake up during the night sometimes thinking about her and many of those times, I find out that she was having a bad night. We were very connected before but now I think we are even more connected.

I carry heavy sadness sometimes when I allow myself to think about what RSD means for Katie now and the uncertainty of what the future holds for her. She is in her early 30's and should be enjoying the normal life of a 30 year old. She is afraid to bring someone else into this life that she is now living. I tell her that she can't make that choice for another person. I continue to pray that she will allow herself the chance to fall in love, and let someone fall in love with her, RSD and all.

I find the strength and courage to help her deal with RSD because that is what I can do. Her Dad and I help as much as we can physically and emotionally to support her. Fortunately, we live close to each other. But hers is a day to day, sometimes hour to hour struggle. We cherish her "good" days and walk through the bad days with the hope that tomorrow will be better. But I worry for her as time goes on. What does her future hold? What other wicked turn will RSD make? And, who will be there for her when her Dad and I are no longer able?

Katie has had to handle difficult decisions, health care choices, as well as deal with the bureaucracies of workers compensation. Her strength and her courage to face each day and each new turn that RSD takes, continues to amaze me. She is an incredible young woman who is determined not to let RSD dictate the person that she is. I am so very proud of her and humbled by her courage and determination and so very grateful that she is my daughter.

Looking For A Needle In The Haystack Only To Find A Piece Of Hay In A Thousand Needles.
A Mother's Story

Danielle has an incredible gift of assisting others to over come their fears and challenges using her four legged friends, her horses. She believes that the greatest things you fear in life are usually the most worthwhile.

Danielle wakes up every day in more pain than most will feel in their lifetime. Her pain which is also known as full body CRPS or RSD, keeps her most days from doing what she most enjoys, spending time with her horses. She is limited in her ability to care for them and her ability to ride for short and the long hours she once did because it is just too painful.

When she was just 13 years old, she created a program which she named, From Fear to Freedom. Her program assisted many people, the youngest being 5 to the eldest participant being 68, in overcoming their fear of riding horses. Many had been bucked off or had some fear of why they wouldn't get in the saddle and enjoy the joy of riding as Danielle did. The program was a tremendous success and she entered and won a grant from Tiger Woods Foundation and Target Stores for $5000.

She continued her work and developed a business at age 15 called Drop Your Reins which was named after her signature move, which was to stand on the back of a horse while learning to trust yourself and the horse then dropping the horse's reins. It is so graceful to see her and others as they became one with the horse and the freedom they experienced could be seen on their faces. Her business grew and she was being mentored as she took it to international audiences. She was working with ADHD and Autistic children to balance their energy and gain focus.

This all came to a screeching halt when her stomach started having pains that 2 hospitals and many doctors were unable to diagnose. She had symptoms of dizziness and fatigue which increased over time. She underwent exploratory surgery to see if they could locate the root of the problem. She felt victimized when doctors said it was all in her head and there must be some psychological reason for her pain.

Finally a year and half later she bumped her knee where she had previously had knee surgery and the pain that she felt was the all too familiar burning that she always felt in her stomach and was now in both her stomach and lower leg. The pain was diagnosed as RSD by an orthopedic after he witnessed the color and temperature changes. She underwent ten days in the hospital and left to scream for 6 days while the psychiatrists put her on major anti convulsants and psychotic medicines which left her in a zombie like state. She was not given anything to cut the pain because they did not believe in giving children with RSD pain medication. On the pain scale RSD/CRPS is the highest and most intense pain a person can have but yet she was left to suffer in several hospitals with over 30 doctors in 2 different states lacking the knowledge to help her until it has spread to her spine and affecting her central nervous system.

At a University Hospital in Florida the staff called in Child Protection Team and Children and Family Services and investigated the entire family for child abuse. Their world began to turn upside down and spiral in what would be the first of many negative experiences that their family would have with the medical community. They whisked Danielle's mother I off to a separate room to be interrogated like a criminal in a police investigation while the Child Protection Doctor terrorized and hurt Danielle. The CP doctor was clearly there on her own agenda and not one to support and help Danielle. The doctor grabbed Danielle's burning RSD/CRPS leg, held it down causing Danielle excruciating pain and made threats to Danielle that if she did not cut this out they would throw her in a psych ward. She said they would take her away from her family. Danielle and her mother came to the hospital to get help and left fearing the ones who were supposed to help find some kind of solution.

Danielle's body was undergoing so many changes with new symptoms such as bladder retention, uncontrollable vomiting, depression, anxiety out of no where, insomnia, and her pain continued to be relentless.

We began traveling in search of answers and new treatments for her symptoms. They went up to the northeast in desperate search to find Danielle some relief. The Calamare Therapy which they sought to relieve her symptoms made Danielle's body react in increased pain. I took Danielle to the emergency room to find help because she could not fly home with her in the current state and unbearable symptoms. They soon discovered the same patterns of the pediatric medical community in Rhode Island that we had experienced in Florida. They treated our family with skepticism and cruelty. Danielle heard people whispering and talking negatively about her and at a young age of 15 she was scared to death.

I had two daughter's to care for and we were thousands of miles away from any family and friends. She was alone to make decisions, juggle her ability to interact with the medical teams, be with Danielle and then also ensure my 7 year old daughter Leila's emotional and development was not affected too much by what our family was enduring.

On the second day of hospitalization in the Rhode Island pediatric hospital, My time was being pulled in two directions. I needed to check in on Leila who was having to spend many hours amusing herself in the playroom by herself because of Danielle's endless screams of pain in her room. It was too much for anyone to handle much less a little sister. I stepped out of Danielle's room and she went into a panic. She needed her mom. She was hurting and scared to death. Danielle got into her wheel chair and screamed down the halls looking for me in a panic. Her body's central nervous system was in the full flight and fight mode. There was nothing she could have done to control it. It was in hyper drive like a rocket taking off into orbit. Danielle rolled towards the elevators looking for me She pushed the button and the nurses along with security guards snatched her up, took her back to her room with Danielle kicking and screaming because of the pain. She just wanted her mom. She was slammed into her bed and handcuffed with leather restrains. When she got loose, the young macho guards grabbed her on her RSD burning legs and slapped her with the leather straps. They then pierced her with a needle full of medicine to sedate her. All of this could have been avoided if they would have thought to get me.

After that our family's ability to visit with Danielle was monitored and I was only allowed to see Danielle an hour a day. They did not give Danielle medicines to relieve her pain and left her screaming for 8 more days. Her sympathetic nervous system was driving and the more it was left to run the show, the more pain Danielle was enduring.
The girls and were still in RI for Christmas. Leila had made many handmade Christmas decorations during the many hours she was alone. I, trying to make the best of the

situation. went to Walgreens late Christmas Eve with Leila. I wanted to make Christmas as special as I could. I asked the manager if he had any trees left for me to decorate in my daughter's hospital room. He donated a beautiful 5 foot tall artificial tree for us to decorate. Leila assisted me in putting the tree together in the hallway of the hospital at 10 PM while Danielle slept. We wanted Danielle to wake up the next morning and for all of them to share their love together in spite of their circumstances. Danielle awoke on Christmas morning to a tree surrounded by gifts donated by Ronald Mc Donald House and friends and family back home. The girls were beginning to open their presents when the doctor came in and spoiled the party. She demanded that Leila and I would have to follow her plan and could only visit with Danielle one hour. We were all crushed and saddened. Christmas Day came to a crashing halt when Danielle tried to convey to the doctor that it was not her mom and sister that were the problem... it was her RSD/CRPS.

I then tried to sign my daughter out of the hospital and take her home. I was advised and threatened that I could not do so. Danielle was under a constant guard 24/7 since the elevator incident. Scared to death with men sitting guard watching over her all night while they flirted and gossiped with the nurses just added fuel to the fire for Danielle. I did not know how to help or protect her daughter from the people who were supposed to be helping her so I started reaching out. I had to make phone calls to RSDSA and have them intercede. A psych evaluation was ordered and Danielle passed with flying colors. She was finally released and discharged from the hospital after 10 days of hell.
Danielle, Leila, and I, all suffered lasting effects from the post traumatic trauma they experienced. Leila to this day, will run if she hears a video of her sister's screams. It will take her right back to that time when all she wanted was them to help get her old sister back.

In 2012, after three years on the journey, once again we sought a new doctor in South Florida in hopes of getting one of the only treatment that has shown promising results for calming the burning pain, Ketamine. Before the doctor would administer the infusion he made Danielle be evaluated by his neuropsychologist and only him. I drove Danielle down to Miami to the doctor in the middle of a tropical storm because we had waited 3 months for the appointment. Because we were desperate we took dangerous risks and made the trip. We faced danger head on because what did we have to loose. So we thought.

Months after the evaluation, Danielle was hospitalized because of another tropical storm which sent her autonomic system into crisis. She could not catch up to the rapid changes in the weather. The doctors were trying to help her until her insurance company gave her current doctor the report from the neuropsychologist. The report was so inaccurate. He based his report on other doctors reports in the past and not on his own findings. He reported over 30 inaccurate statements in his report with the most damaging was that, " Danielle was muchausen by proxy and that it was suggested that Danielle was making it up." He also stated, " It was his belief that I was a huge factor and that I was getting secondary gains and benefits from her interaction with the medical community." In his report he diagnosed Danielle with Factilios which is the new word for muchausen disease where the patient causes harm to themselves to gain attention.

All her doctors began withholding treatment and questioning everything. Instead of helping me find relief for Danielle once again they put a guard on Danielle and watched her every move. They discontinued the ketamine treatments that Danielle had been searching over a year for a doctor to administer. She was sent home with barely any medication and because she was almost 19, the doctor started transitioning her out of his care. All this because of a falsified report that an unqualified doctor made which poisoned the minds of a team that was trying to help her.

Danielle and our entire family has suffered at the hands of many they sought for help in the medical community. The system is an institution designed to operated in fear rather than compassion and love. Accusations have caused more hurt and pain for Danielle especially psychologically and emotionally. She has always been a good girl and it seems they are trying hard to make her out to be a bad one. She is just a young girl whose life was dramatically changed along with our families. When her body's central nervous system went haywire and caused her to have dysautonomia – imbalance of the autonomic nervous system.

Every new road ended up being a dead end. We thought they saw the light at the end of the tunnel with the hope of a cure or something or someone to relieve Danielle's pain but it always turned out to be only a mirage. An illusion. Another needle in the haystack.
Unknowing what the future holds, Danielle has days where she wants to just give up because she looses sight of knowing a life without pain so she can enjoy the things in life that bring her joy. She no longer can help others in over coming their fears because she is faced with the overwhelming guilt that she is burdening everyone she loves with her painful existence.

As Plato's quote reminds us, "Be kind, for everyone you meet is fighting a hard battle." We never know what the battle might be because most inflicted with RSD/CRPS look fine on the outside while their bodies are raging infernos on the inside
.
Danielle, her little sister Leila and I are inspiring people still with their courage and strength. It is their hope that people will learn to set aside their judgments of one another and begin to treat others with love and compassion. They also wish to inspire people to look for their blessings no matter how small because that is what can carry you forward in the most difficult of time.
FInd Your Piece of Hay.

APPENDIX A
Social Security Ruling:

"[Federal Register: October 20, 2003 (Volume 68, Number 202)/Notices]
[Page 59971–59976]
EFFECTIVE DATE: October 20, 2003
Policy Interpretation Ruling
Titles II and XVI: Evaluating Cases Involving Reflex Sympathetic Dystrophy Syndrome/Complex Regional Pain Syndrome

Purpose:
To explain the policies of the Social Security Administration for developing and evaluating title II and title XVI claims for disability on the basis of Reflex Sympathetic Dystrophy Syndrome (RSDS), also frequently known as Complex Regional Pain Syndrome, Type I (CRPS). These terms are synonymous and are used to describe a unique clinical syndrome that may develop following trauma. This syndrome is characterized by complaints of intense pain and typically includes signs of autonomic dysfunction.
Citations (Authority):
Sections 216(i), 223(d), 1614(a)(3), 1614(a)(4) and 1614(c) of the Social Security Act (the Act), as amended; Regulations No. 4, subpart P, sections 404.1502, 404.1505, 404.1508–404.1509, 404.1511–404.1513, 404.1520, 404.1520a, 404.1521, 404.1523, 404.1526–404.1530, 404.1545–404.1546, 404.1560–404.1569a; and 404.1593–404.1594 and appendix 1; and Regulations No. 16, subpart I, sections 416.902, 416.905, 416.906, 416.908–416.909, 416.911–416.913, 416.920, 416.920a, 416.921, 416.923, 416.924, 416.924a-416.924c, 416.925, 416.926, 416.926a, 416.927–416.930, 416.945–416.946, 416.960–416.969a, 416.987, and 416.993–416.994a.
Introduction:

RSDS/CRPS are terms used to describe a constellation of symptoms and signs that may occur following an injury to bone or soft tissue. The precipitating injury may be so minor that the individual does not even recall sustaining an injury. Other potential precipitants suggested by the medical literature include, but are not limited to, surgical procedures, drug exposure, stroke with hemiplegia, and cervical spondylosis.

Policy Interpretation
What Is RSDS/CRPS?
RSDS/CRPS is a chronic pain syndrome most often resulting from trauma to a single extremity. It can also result from diseases, surgery, or injury affecting other parts of the body. Even a minor injury can trigger RSDS/CRPS. The most common acute clinical manifestations include complaints of intense pain and findings indicative of autonomic dysfunction at the site of the precipitating trauma. Later, spontaneously occurring pain may be associated with abnormalities in the affected region involving the skin, subcutaneous tissue, and bone. It is characteristic of this syndrome that the degree of pain reported is out of proportion to the severity of the injury sustained by the individual. When left untreated, the signs and symptoms of the disorder may worsen over time.

Although the pathogenesis of this disorder (the precipitating mechanism(s) of the signs and symptoms characteristic of RSDS/CRPS) has not been defined, dysfunction of the sympathetic nervous system has been strongly implicated.

The sympathetic nervous system regulates the body's involuntary physiological responses to stressful stimuli. Sympathetic stimulation results in physiological changes that prepare the body to respond to a stressful stimulus by "fight or flight." The so-called "fight or flight" response is characterized by constriction of peripheral vasculature (blood vessels supplying skin), increase in heart rate and sweating, dilatation of bronchial tubes, dilatation of pupils, increase in level of alertness, and constriction of sphincter musculature.

Abnormal sympathetic nervous system function may produce inappropriate or exaggerated neural signals that may be misinterpreted as pain. In addition, abnormal sympathetic stimulation may produce changes in blood vessels, skin, musculature and bone. Early recognition of the syndrome and prompt treatment, ideally within 3 months of the first symptoms, provides the greatest opportunity for effective recovery.

How Does RSDS/CRPS Typically Present?
RSDS/CRPS patients typically report persistent, burning, aching or searing pain that is initially localized to the site of the injury. The involved area usually has increased sensitivity to touch. The degree of reported pain is often out of proportion to the severity of the precipitating injury. Without appropriate treatment, the pain and associated atrophic skin and bone changes may spread to involve an entire limb. Cases have been reported to progress and spread to other limbs, or to remote parts of the body.
Clinical studies have demonstrated that when treatment is delayed, the signs and symptoms may progress and spread, resulting in long-term and even permanent physical and psychological problems. Some investigators have found that the signs and symptoms of RSDS/CRPS persist longer than 6 months in 50 percent of cases, and may last for years in cases where treatment is not successful.

What Are the Diagnostic Criteria for RSDS/CRPS?
A diagnosis of RSDS/CRPS requires the presence of complaints of persistent, intense pain that results in impaired mobility of the affected region. The complaints of pain are associated with:

Swelling;
Autonomic instability—seen as changes in skin color or texture, changes in sweating (decreased or excessive sweating), skin temperature changes, or abnormal pilomotor erection (gooseflesh);

Abnormal hair or nail growth (growth can be either too slow or too fast);

Osteoporosis; or Involuntary movements of the affected region of the initial injury.

Progression of the clinical disorder is marked by worsening of a previously identified finding, or the manifestation of additional abnormal changes in the skin, nails, muscles, joints, ligaments, and bones of the affected region. Clinical progression does not necessarily correlate with specific timeframes. Efficacy of treatment must be judged on the basis of the treatment's effect on the pain and whether or not progressive changes continue in the tissues of the affected region.

Reported pain at the site of the injury may be followed by complaints of muscle pain, joint stiffness, restricted mobility, or abnormal hair and nail growth in the affected region. Further, signs of autonomic instability (changes in the color or temperature of the skin and frequent appearance of goose bumps) may develop in the affected region. Osteoporosis may be noted by appropriate medically acceptable imaging techniques. Complaints of pain can further intensify, and can be reported to spread to involve other extremities. Muscle atrophy and contractures can also develop. Persistent clinical progression resulting in muscle atrophy and contractures, or progression of complaints of pain to include other extremities or regions, in spite of appropriate diagnosis and treatment, hallmark a poor prognosis.

How Is RSDS/CRPS Treated?
Patient education and activity programs designed to increase limb mobility and promote use of the extremity or affected region during activities of daily living are considered the most important treatments for RSDS/CRPS. The medical literature has demonstrated that individuals affected by RSDS/CRPS have a better prognosis when they receive an early diagnosis and mobility is immediately encouraged. In some patients, it is necessary to inject a

long-acting anesthetic to block sympathetic activity and reduce pain to allow the individual to increase the mobility of the affected region. Various analgesics, including narcotics and neurostimulators, may be used to minimize pain and promote the individual's ability to tolerate greater mobility.

A mental evaluation may be requested by treating or other medical sources to determine if any undiagnosed psychiatric disease is present that could potentially contribute to a reduced pain tolerance. It is important to recognize that such evaluations are not based on concern that RSDS/CRPS findings are imaginary or etiologically linked to psychiatric disease. The behavioral and cognitive effects of the medications used to treat pain need to be thoroughly considered in the evaluation of this syndrome.
Other types of medications may also be used to reduce pain. Anti- inflammatory preparations, psychotropic medications (for example, antidepressants), certain antiepileptic drugs, muscle relaxants, and drugs that produce generalized reduction in sympathetic outflow may be tried in an effort to reduce the signs and symptoms associated with RSDS/CRPS and improve the mobility of the affected region.

Patients who are noted to have a good response to local sympathetic blocks may be considered candidates for surgical sympathectomy. This procedure permanently disrupts the sympathetic innervation of the affected region. It involves destroying a sympathetic ganglion and must be performed by a physician who is an expert in this technique. This procedure is not without risk of post-surgical complications.

What Is a Medically Determinable Impairment?
Sections 216(i) and 1614(a)(3) of the Act define "disability"[1] as the inability to engage in any substantial gainful activity by reason of any medically determinable physical or mental impairment (or combination of impairments) which can be expected to result in death or which has lasted or can be expected to last for a continuous

period of not less than 12 months.[2]

Sections 223(d)(3) and 1614(a)(3)(D) of the Act, and 20 CFR 404.1508 and 416.908, require that impairment result from anatomical, physiological, or psychological abnormalities that can be shown by medically acceptable clinical and laboratory diagnostic techniques. The Act and regulations further require that impairment be established by medical evidence that consists of signs, symptoms, and laboratory findings, and not only by an individual's statement of symptoms.

How Is RSDS/CRPS Identified as a Medically Determinable Impairment?

RSDS/CRPS constitutes a medically determinable impairment when it is documented by appropriate medical signs, symptoms, and laboratory findings, as discussed above. RSDS/CRPS may be the basis for a finding of "disability." Disability may not be established on the basis of an individual's statement of symptoms alone.

For purposes of Social Security disability evaluation, RSDS/CRPS can be established in the presence of persistent complaints of pain that are typically out of proportion to the severity of any documented precipitant and one or more of the following clinically documented signs in the affected region at any time following the documented precipitant:

Swelling;

Autonomic instability—seen as changes in skin color or texture, changes in sweating (decreased or excessive sweating), changes in skin temperature, and abnormal pilomotor erection (gooseflesh);

Abnormal hair or nail growth (growth can be either too slow or too fast);

Osteoporosis; or Involuntary movements of the affected region of the initial injury.

When longitudinal treatment records document persistent limiting pain in an area where one or more of these abnormal signs has been documented at some point in time since the date of the precipitating injury, disability adjudicators can reliably determine that RSDS/CRPS is present and constitutes a medically determinable impairment. It may be noted in the treatment records that these signs are not present continuously, or the signs may be present at one examination and not appear at another. Transient findings are characteristic of RSDS/CRPS, and do not affect a finding that a medically determinable impairment is present.

How Is Medical Evidence of the Impairment Documented?
In cases involving RSDS/CRPS, the documentation of medical signs or laboratory findings at some point in time in the clinical record since the date of the precipitating injury is critical in establishing the presence of a medically determinable impairment. In cases in which RSDS/CRPS is alleged, longitudinal clinical records reflecting ongoing medical evaluation and treatment from the individual's medical sources, especially treating sources, are extremely helpful in documenting the presence of any medical signs, symptoms and laboratory findings.

Generally, evidence for the 12-month period preceding the month of application should be obtained, unless there is reason to believe that development of an earlier period is necessary, the alleged onset of disability is less than 12 months before the date of the application, or a fully favorable determination can be made with less evidence.
If the adjudicator finds that the evidence is inadequate to determine whether the individual is disabled, he or she must first recontact the individual's treating or other medical source(s) to determine whether the additional information needed is readily available, in accordance with 20 CFR 404.1512 and 416.912. Only after the adjudicator determines that the information is not readily available from the individual's health care provider(s), or that the necessary information or clarification cannot be sought from the individual's health care provider(s), should the adjudicator proceed to arrange for a consultative examination(s) in accordance with 20 CFR 404.1519a and 416.919a. The type of consultative examination(s) purchased will depend on the nature of the individual's symptoms and the extent of the

evidence already in the case record.

It should be noted that conflicting evidence in the medical record is not unusual in cases of RSDS due to the transitory nature of its objective findings and the complicated diagnostic process involved. Clarification of any such conflicts in the medical evidence should be sought first from the individual's treating or other medical sources.

Medical opinions from treating sources about the nature and severity of an individual's impairment(s) are entitled to deference and may be entitled to controlling weight. If we find that a treating source's medical opinion on the issue of the nature and severity of an individual's impairment(s) is well–supported by medically acceptable clinical and laboratory diagnostic techniques and is not inconsistent with the other substantial evidence in the case record, the adjudicator will give it controlling weight. (See SSR 96-2p, "Titles II and XVI: Giving Controlling Weight to Treating Source Medical Opinions," and SSR 96-5p, "Titles II and XVI: Medical Source Opinions on Issues Reserved to the Commissioner.")[3]

How Is the Duration and Severity of RSDS/CRPS Established?
The signs and symptoms of RSDS/CRPS may remain stable over time, improve, or worsen. Documentation should, whenever appropriate, include a longitudinal clinical record containing detailed medical observations, treatment, the individual's response to treatment, complications of treatment, and a detailed description of how the impairment limits the individual's ability to function and perform or sustain work activity over time.
Chronic pain and many of the medications prescribed to treat it may affect an individual's ability to maintain attention and concentration, as well as adversely affect his or her cognition, mood, and behavior, and may even reduce motor reaction times. These factors can interfere with an individual's ability to sustain work activity over time, or preclude sustained work activity altogether. When evaluating duration and severity, as well as when evaluating RFC, the effects of chronic pain and the use of pain

medications must be carefully considered.

When the alleged onset of disability secondary to RSDS/ CRPS occurred less than 12 months before adjudication, the adjudicator must evaluate the available medical evidence and project the degree of impairment severity that is likely to exist at the end of 12 months. Information about treatment and response to treatment, as well as any medical source opinions about the individual's prognosis at the end of 12 months, are helpful in deciding whether the medically determinable impairment is expected to be of disabling severity for at least 12 consecutive months.

In those cases in which an individual is found disabled based on RSDS/CRPS, but medical improvement is anticipated, the adjudicator should schedule an appropriate medical reexamination date consistent with the information indicating the likelihood of medical improvement.

How Is RSDS/CRPS Evaluated?

Claims in which the individual alleges RSDS/CRPS are adjudicated using the sequential evaluation process, just as for any other impairment. Because finding that RSDS/CRPS is a medically determinable impairment requires the presence of chronic pain and one or more clinically documented signs in the affected region, the adjudicator can reliably find that pain is an expected symptom in this disorder. Other symptoms, including such things as extreme sensitivity to touch or pressure, or abnormal sensations of heat or cold, can also be associated with this disorder. Given that a variety of symptoms can be associated with RSDS/CRPS, once the disorder has been established as a medically determinable impairment, the adjudicator must evaluate the intensity, persistence, and limiting effects of the individual's symptoms to determine the extent to which the symptoms limit the individual's ability to do basic work activities. For this purpose, whenever the individual's statements about the intensity, persistence, or functionally limiting effects of pain or other symptoms are not substantiated by objective medical evidence, the adjudicator must make a finding on the credibility of the individual's statements based on a consideration of the entire case record. This includes the medical signs and laboratory findings, the individual's own statements about the symptoms, any statements and other information provided by treating or examining physicians or psychologists and other persons about the symptoms and how they affect the individual, and any other relevant evidence in the case record. Although symptoms alone cannot be the basis for finding a medically determinable impairment, once the existence of a medically determinable impairment has been established, an individual's symptoms and the effect(s) of those symptoms on the individual's ability to function must be considered both in determining impairment severity and in assessing the individual's residual functional capacity (RFC), as appropriate. If the adjudicator finds that pain or other symptoms cause a limitation or restriction having more than a minimal effect on an individual's ability to perform basic work activities, a "severe" impairment must be found to exist. See SSR 96–3p, "Titles II and XVI:

APPENDIX B
MEDICAL RECORDS REQUEST FORM

Medical Records Request Form:

Your name
Your address
Your phone number and Fax number if applicable

Doctor's/hospital's name
Doctor's/hospital's address
Fax #
Attn: Medical Records

Date

Dear Medical Records Dept:

I am hereby giving you permission to release my medical records from (date) to (date). Please be sure to including all tests, nurses notes, procedures, and doctor's notes. Please send them to me at the above address. My date of birth is:

(If your records are in a different name be sure to put that after your date of birth. I was a patient under the name of:)

Sincerely,

APPENDIX C
Codes for CRPS/RSD
ICD 9 AND ICD 10 CODES

355.9 Mononeuritis of unspecified site
Causalgia NOS
Complex regional pain syndrome NOS
Excludes:
causalgia:
lower limb (355.71)
upper limb (354.4)
complex regional pain syndrome:
lower limb (355.71)
upper limb (354.4)

354.4 Causalgia of upper limb
Complex regional pain syndrome type II of the upper limb
Excludes:
causalgia:
NOS (355.9)
lower limb (355.71)
complex regional pain syndrome type II of the lower limb
(355.71)

337.20 Reflex sympathetic dystrophy, unspecified
Complex regional pain syndrome type I, unspecified

337.29 Reflex sympathetic dystrophy of other specified site
Complex regional pain syndrome type I of other specified
site

337.21 Reflex sympathetic dystrophy of the upper limb
Complex regional pain syndrome type I of the upper limb

337.22 Reflex sympathetic dystrophy of the lower limb
Complex regional pain syndrome type I of the lower limb

355.71 Causalgia of lower limb
Excludes:
causalgia:
NOS (355.9)
upper limb (354.4)
complex regional pain syndrome type II of the upper limb
(354.4)

ICD 10 CODES FOR CRPS (RSDS) – INTERNATIONAL DISEASE
CODES
Here are the ICD 10 Codes, to replace the current ICD 9
Codes (ICD = International Disease Codes). These codes are
supposed to be used by Drs around the world to help
differentiate between the various types of CRPS.

G90.5 Complex regional pain syndrome I (CRPS I)
REFLEX SYMPATHETIC DYSTROPHY

Excludes: causalgia of lower limb (G57.7)
Causalgia of upper limb (G56.4)
Complex regional pain syndrome II of lower limb (G57.7)
Complex regional pain syndrome II of upper limb (G56.4)

G90.50 Complex regional pain syndrome, unspecified
G90.51 Complex regional pain syndrome of upper limb
G90.511 Complex regional pain syndrome of right upper
limb

G90.512 Complex regional pain syndrome of left upper
limb

G90.513 Complex regional pain syndrome of upper limb,
bilateral

G90.519 Complex regional pain syndrome of unspecified
upper limb

G90.52 Complex regional pain syndrome of lower limb

G90.521 Complex regional pain syndrome of right lower limb

G90.522 Complex regional pain syndrome of left lower limb

G90.523 Complex regional pain syndrome of lower limb, bilateral

G90.529 Complex regional pain syndrome of unspecified lower limb

G90.59 Complex regional pain syndrome of other specified site

INTERNATIONAL DISEASE CODES FOR RSDS – (these are the old Codes)
International Disease Code Numbers assigned to the various types of RSD;

337.20 Unspecified site
337.21 Upper Extremity
337.22 Lower Extremity
337.29 Other Specified Site

IV Ketamine Codes (In Patient & Out Patient Codes)
Ketamine Billing Codes for Insurance Coverage

Codes for outpatient: IV Ketamine Outpatient Codes / Lidocaine Outpatient Codes
Code Item:
99213 Outpatient E&M Established Patient
96365 IV Infusion therapy/P
96366 IVInfusion therapy P
36000 Intro Needle/Intracat
93041 Rhythm ECG 1–3 leads
J3490 Ketamine, IV
J2405 Ondansetron HCL Injection
J2765 Metoclopramide HCL Injection
J2250 Injection Midazolam Hydroch
J7030 Infusion Normal Saline
J2001 – Intravenous infusion of IV Lidocaine

INPATIENT Codes (I don't have the codes for the lab work as that varies from doctor to doctor but their will be daily lab work) IV Ketamine inpatient codes / Lidocaine

Code Item Day
99223 Initial Hospital Services Level 3 H&P Day 1
99255 Level 5 Hospital Consult Day 1
90760 Intravenous infusion, hydration; initial, 31 minutes to 1 hour Day 1
99295 Initial Inpatient, Intensive Care Unit, Room & Board, Incidentals Day 1
76499 Chest X-Ray Reading Day 2
99233 Level 3 Progress Note Day 2
99222 Level 3 Progress Note Day 3
99255 Level 5 Hospital Consult Day 3
99252 Level 2 Hospital Consult Day 4
99255 Level 5 Hospital Consult Day 4
99233 Level 3 Progress Note Day 5
99252 Level 2 Hospital Consult Day 5
99233 Level 3 Progress Note Day 6
99255 Level 5 Hospital Consult Day 6
99255 Level 5 Hospital Consult Day 7
Lab Services Day 1–7

90761 Intravenous infusion, hydration; each additional hour (List separately in addition to code for primary procedure)

Day 1–7
90774 Therapeutic, prophylactic or diagnostic injection (specify substance or drug); intravenous push, single or initial substance/drug Day 1–7
99295 Inpatient, Intensive Care Unit, Room& Board, Incidentals, Subsequent Care Day 1–7
J3490 Unclassified drug (use for Ketamine) Day 1–7
J2001 – Intravenous infusion of IV Lidocaine

APPENDIX D
THE MEDICATION PUMP

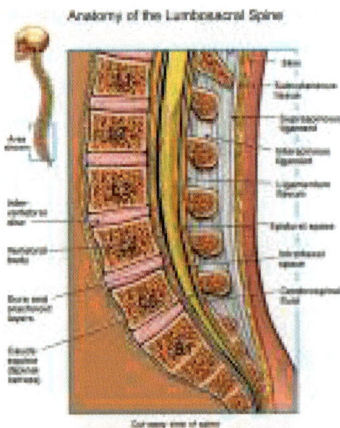

The above photo illustrates where the catheter is placed in the spine. With this implanted devise a small pump, about the size of a hockey puck is placed in the lower abdomen. A catheter is tunneled under the skin and placed into the intrathecal space in the spinal column.

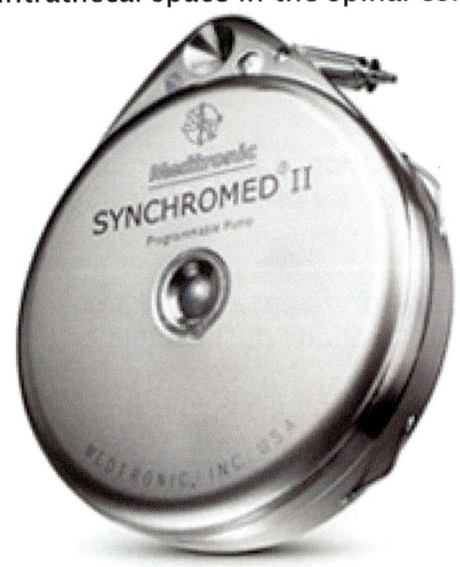

A battery is contained within the pump as well as a reservoir that can contain medications. The pump pushes the medication through the catheter into the intrathecal space in your spine where it is dispersed and bathes the spinal cord.

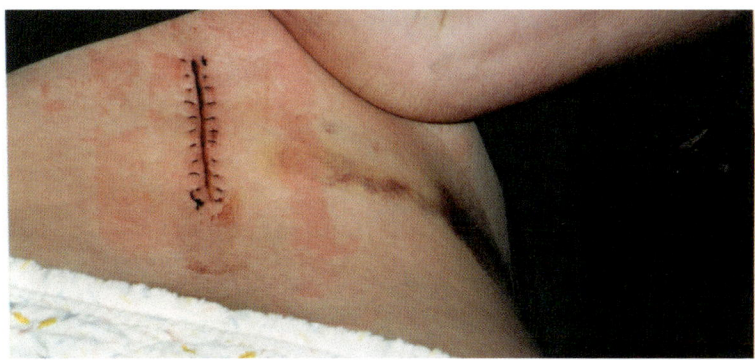

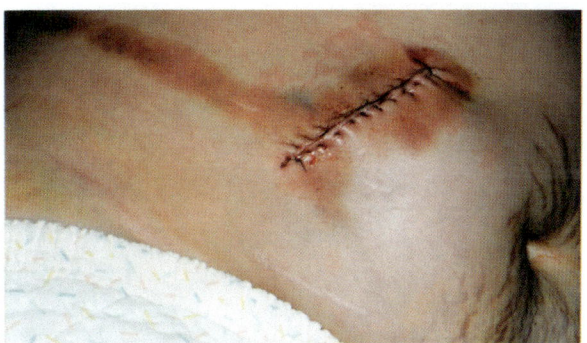

Once the sutures are out and the incisions are healed, the pump can be used. The pump has a reservoir that can be filled with medications. Narcotics, such as Morphine can be placed into the pump as can anti-spasmodic medications such as Baclofen or a combination of medications. Many people with RSD have dystonia. Baclofen in a medication pump can offer them great relief from the dystonia because it delivers continuous medication at a steady rate right into the spinal fluid.

The pump is programed via radio frequency with a wand placed externally over the pump by a specially trained nurse and doctor. The pump is refilled by a specially trained nurse or doctor. I have photos of my Medtronic (the manufacturer of my pump) being refilled back in 2000.

First the area over the pump is cleaned with betadine to clean any germs off of the skin and prevent them from being introduced into the pump when the needle is inserted. Here you can see my nurse cleaning my abdomen with the betadine solution.

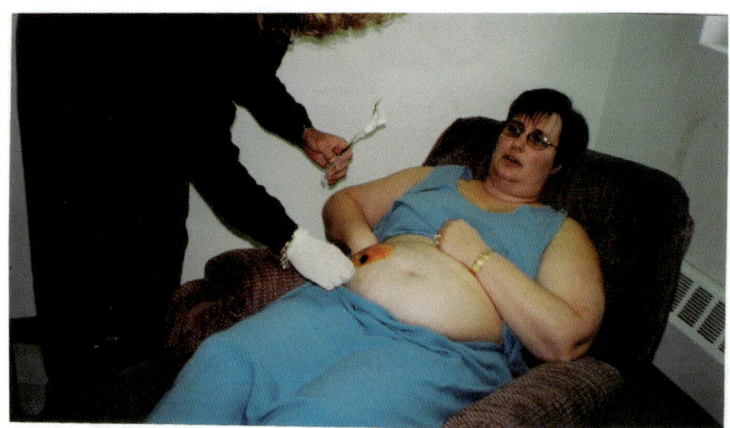

Then a template is placed over the pump. This shows the practitioner exactly where the place on the pump is that the needle should be placed. A sterile drape is placed over my abdomen. The drape has a hole in it for the template.

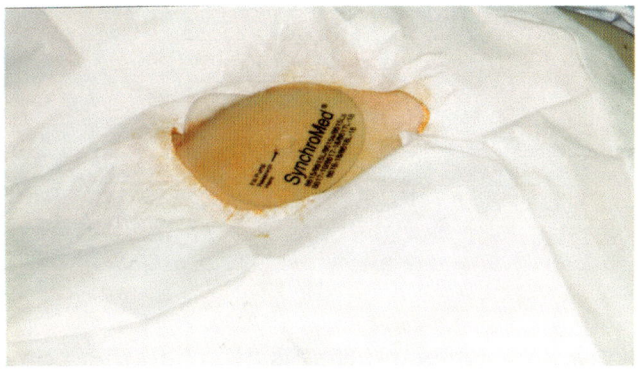

Once the template is in place, the practitioner feels for the edges of the pump and aligns the template along the edges of the pump so that they match up. The syringe is filled with the proper mix of medication, attached to a filter, tubing and a special needle. The template shows the practitioner exactly where the reservoir is in the.

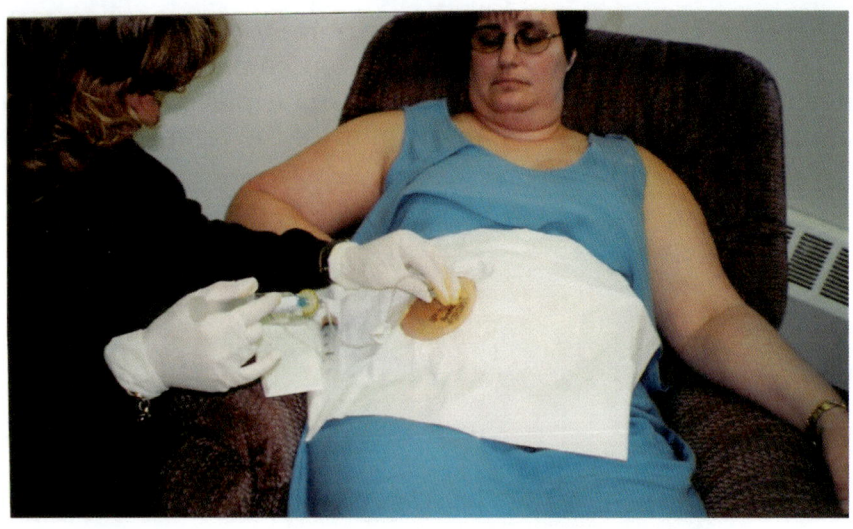

Using a radio wave wand that is attached to a computer, the practitioner can program the pump to infuse the medication into the intrathecal space as prescribed by the doctor.

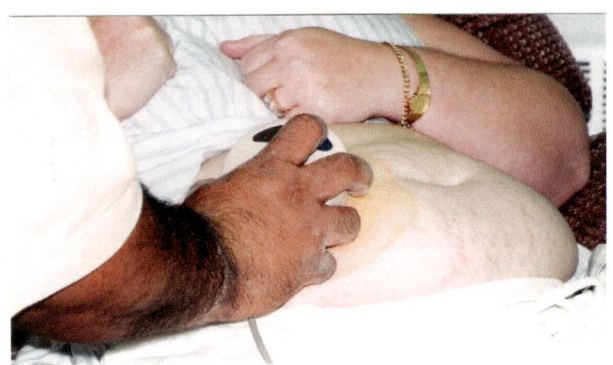

APPENDIX E
SUICIDE HOTLINE INFORMATION

The suicide rate among those with RSD is high. If you are feeling suicidal, pick up the phone and make a call to the Suicide & Crisis Hotline.

www.suicidehotlines.com is a web site that lets you know what the call will be like. You can call, chat, go to web sites, email or call the crisis hot lines. Here are two numbers that you can call:

HOPE
1-800-SUICIDE
(1-800-784-2433)

The National Suicide Prevention Lifeline:
1-800-273-TALK
(1-800-273-0355)

Help is just on the other side of the phone line where you will find professionals who will help with words of comfort to those in crisis. They can direct you to health care professionals in your area.

APPENDIX F
SECTION 504

Section 504 of the Debilitation Act is a civil rights law. It prohibits discrimination against individuals with disabilities and ensures that a child with a disability, e.g. RSD/CRPS, has equal access to an education. The portion of Section 504 of the Rehabilitation Act at 29 U. S. C 794 states:

Section 794. Nondiscrimination Under Federal Grants and Programs Promulgation of nondiscriminatory rules and regulations. No otherwise qualified individual with a disability in the United States, as defined in Sec. 705(20) of this title, shall, solely by reason of her or his disability, be excluded from the participation in, be denied the benefits of, or be subjected to discrimination under any program or activity receiving Federal financial assistance or under any program or activity conducted by any Executive agency or by the United States Postal Service...

Section 504 protects all persons with a disability who have:
* a physical or mental impairment that substantially limits one or more major life activities

*Have a record of such an impairment

*Are regarded as having such impairment

Under Section 504, a child may receive accommodations and modifications of his/her impairment substantially limits the ability to learn. Children with RSD/CRPS may be entitled to special services under the Individuals with Disabilities Education Act (IDEA). IDEA requires the school to provide an individualized educational program (IEP) that is designated to meet the child's unique needs and provides the child with educational benefit. Fewer procedural saguaros are available for disabled children and their parents under Section 504 than under IDEA.

APPENDIX G
LINKS TO ARTICLES ON CRPS/RSD

This is a listing of articles from several reputable scientific journals and web sites. It does not represent all of the information on CRPS/RSD or the opinion of the author of this book. It is a sampling of the research that can be found on line.

Dental Care and Chronic Pain
www.rsds.org/3/treatment/Siegelman_Denistry/html

Chronic Pain Rehabilitation Program
http://my.clevelandclinic.org/chronic_pain/default.aspx?utm_campaign=cprp-url&utm_medium=offline&utm_source=redirect

Deconstructing Complex Regional Pain Syndrome
http://www.practicalpainmanagement.com/pain/neuropathic/crps/deconstructing-complex-regional-pain-syndrome

Intra-nasal Low Dose Ketamine
http://painmuse.org/?p=329

http://www.rsds.org/pdfsall/Webster_Walker.pdf

Remission in Sympathetically Maintained RSD
http://www.rsds.org/Research_Articles/Lesley_Mazloomdoost_Agarwal.html

Glia Cell Research:
http://www.rsds.org/3/education/glial%20conference%20summary.html

Emergency Room Protocols for RSD
http://www.rsdsa.org/pdfsall/Emergency-protocol-final.pdf

Hospital Protocol for RSD
http://www.rsdsa.org/pdfsall/hospital_protocol.pdf

Aquatherapy
http://www.rsdhope.org/aqua-therapy.html

Medications
http://www.rsdhope.org/medication-articles.html

Chronic Pain Rehabilitation Program
http://my.clevelandclinic.org/chronic_pain/default.aspx?
utm_campaign=cprp-
url&utm_medium=offline&utm_source=redirect

Credible RSD Organizations:
www.rsdsa.org
www.rsdhope.org
www.forgrace.org
www.crpspartnersinpain.com

Some articles on Lidocaine infusions are:
www.rsds.org/pdfsall/
SchwartzmanRJ_PatelM_GrothusenJR.pdf

www.rsda.orgpdfall//
maleki.level.bennett.schwartzman.pdf

www.bja.oxfordjournals.org/content/98/2/261.full

Ketamine Articles:

Typical Ketamine Treatment
http://www.rsdsa.org/Treatment/ketamine.html

How to Determine the Effectiveness of Treatments for
RSD / CRPS:
  http://www.rsdfoundation.org/en/en_treatments.html

Typical Ketamine Protocol:
http://www.rsdfoundation.org/en/
ketamine_Treatment.html

What Is Ketamine Infusion Therapy For Complex Regional Pain Syndrome?
http://boneandspine.com/pain-management/what-is-ketamine-infusion-therapy-for-pain/

Ketamine produces effective and long-term pain relief in patients with Complex Regional Pain Syndrome Type 1
http://www.rsds.org/pdfsall/Sigtermans_etal.pdf

Efficacy of Ketamine in Anesthetic Dosage for the Treatment of Refractory Complex Regional Pain Syndrome: An Open-Label Phase II Study
www.rsds.org/pdfsall/Kiefer_Rohr_Ploppa_Dietrich.pdf

The neurocognitive effects of 5 day anesthetic Ketamine for the treatment of refractory complex regional pain syndrome
www.rsds.org/2/library/article_archive/pop/Koffler_Hampstead_Irani%20.pdf

Ketamine produces effective and long-term pain relief in patients with Complex Regional Pain Syndrome Type 1
www.rsds.org/2library/article_archive/pop/Sigtermans_etal.pdf

Dr Getson's Protocol:
http://www.rsds.org/1/publications/review_archive/pdf/Getson_Spring2009.pdf
http://www.ncbi.nlm.nih.gov/pubmed/19783371

Outpatient intravenous ketamine
http://www.ncbi.nlm.nih.gov/pubmed/19783371

Ketamine and Post Traumatic Stress Syndrome:
http://www.ncbi.nlm.nih.gov/pubmed/18376165

The correlation between ketamine and post-traumatic ...
[J Trauma. 2008] – PubMed – NCBI
www.ncbi.nlm.nih.gov

Ketamine and RSD:
http://rsds.org/2/library/article_archive/pop/
ketamine_40.pdf

Overview of Ketamine Infusion Therapy:
http://www.rsds.org/2/library/article_archive/pop/
Schwartzman_Pain2009.pdf

Outpatient Ketamine: A Double Blind Study
http://www.rsdsa.org/Treatment/ketamine.html

How to Determine the Effectiveness of Treatments for
RSD / CRPS
http://www.rsdfoundation.org/en/en_treatments.html

Typical Ketamine Protocol
http://www.rsdfoundation.org/en/
ketamine_Treatment.html

What Is Ketamine Infusion Therapy For Complex Regional
Pain Syndrome?:
http://boneandspine.com/pain-management/what-is-
ketamine-infusion-therapy-for-pain/

Multi-Day Low Dose Ketamine Infusion for the Treatment
of Complex Regional Pain Syndrome
http://www.rsds.org/2/library/article_archive/pop/
goldberg_low_dose_ketamine.pdf

Pathophysiology of Complex Regional Pain Syndrome:
Development of New Treatments:http://www.rsds.org/2/
library/article_archive/pop/
PainPractitionerWinter2007_Schwartzman.html

Update on Low-dose Ketamine Infusions:http://
www.rsds.org/1/publications/review_archive/pdf/
Getson_Spring2009.pdf

Subanesthetic Ketamine Infusion Therapy: A
Retrospective Analysis of a Novel Therapeutic Approach to

Complex Regional Pain Syndrome:
http://www.rsds.org/2/library/article_archive/pop/correll_subanesthetic%20ketamine.pdf

www.who.int/medicines/areas/qualitity_safety/4.3KetamineCriticalReview.pdf

www.ncbi.nlm.nih.gov/pubmed/15109503

Nasal Ketamine Research

Safety and efficacy if intranasal Ketamine for the treatment of breakthrough pain in patients with chronic pain
www.painjournalonline.com/article/S0304-3959(03)00408-1/abstract

European Journal of Pain: Effects of low-dose intranasal (S)-ketamine in patients with neuropathic pain
http://www.rsds.org/pdfsall/Huge_EurJPain_2009.pdf

Safety and Efficacy of Nasal Ketamine
http://www.painjournalonline.com/article/S0304-3959(03)00408-1/abstract

http://www.ncbi.nlm.nih.gov/pubmed/15109503

APPENDIX H
A LETTER FROM DR. ROB ON HOW APPROACH
DOCTORS

A letter from a doctor (Dr. Rob)
Clearly this is a very important issue and this letter touched a nerve that has largely been ignored.

Dear Patients:
You have it very hard, much harder than most people understand. Having sat for 16 years listening to the stories, seeing the tiredness in your eyes, hearing you try to describe the indescribable, I have come to understand that I too can't understand what your lives are like. How do you answer the question, "how do you feel?" when you've forgotten what "normal" feels like? How do you deal with all of the people who think you are exaggerating your pain, your emotions, your fatigue? How do you decide when to believe them or when to trust your own body? How do you cope with living a life that won't let you forget about your frailty, your limits, your mortality?
I can't imagine.

But I do bring something to the table that you may not know. I do have information that you can't really understand because of your unique perspective, your battered world. There is something that you need to understand that, while it won't undo your pain, make your fatigue go away, or lift your emotions, it will help you. It's information without which you bring yourself more pain than you need suffer; it's a truth that is a key to getting the help you need much easier than you have in the past. It may not seem important, but trust me, it is.
You scare doctors.

No, I am not talking about the fear of disease, pain, or death. I am not talking about doctors being afraid of the limits of their knowledge. I am talking about your understanding of a fact that everyone else seems to miss, a fact that many doctors hide from: we are normal, fallible people who happen to doctor for a job. We are not special.

In fact, many of us are very insecure, wanting to feel the affirmation of people who get better, hearing the praise of those we help. We want to cure disease, to save lives, to be the helping hand, the right person in the right place at the right time.

But chronic unsolvable disease stands square in our way. You don't get better, and it makes many of us frustrated, and it makes some of us mad at you. We don't want to face things we can't fix because it shows our limits. We want the miraculous, and you deny us that chance.

And since this is the perspective you have when you see doctors, your view of them is quite different. You see us getting frustrated. You see us when we feel like giving up. When we take care of you, we have to leave behind the illusion of control, of power over disease. We get angry, feel insecure, and want to move on to a patient who we can fix, save, or impress. You are the rock that proves how easily the ship can be sunk. So your view of doctors is quite different.

Then there is the fact that you also possess something that is usually our domain: knowledge. You know more about your disease than many of us do – most of us do. Your MS, rheumatoid arthritis, end–stage kidney disease, Cushing's disease, bipolar disorder, chronic pain disorder, brittle diabetes, or disabling psychiatric disorder – your defining pain –– is something most of us don't regularly encounter. It's something most of us try to avoid. So you possess deep understanding of something that many doctors don't possess. Even doctors who specialize in your disorder don't share the kind of knowledge you can only get through living with a disease. It's like a parent's knowledge of their child versus that of a pediatrician. They may have breadth of knowledge, but you have depth of knowledge that no doctor can possess.

So when you approach a doctor – especially one you've never met before – you come with a knowledge of your disease that they don't have, and a knowledge of the doctor's limitations that few other patients have. You see why you scare doctors? It's not your fault that you do, but ignoring this fact will limit the help you can only get from them. I know this because, just like you know your disease better than any doctor, I know what being a doctor feels like more than any patient could ever understand. You encounter doctors intermittently (more than you wish, perhaps); I live as a doctor continuously.

So let me be so bold as to give you advice on dealing with doctors. There are some things you can do to make things easier, and others that can sabotage any hope of a good relationship:

1.Don't come on too strong – yes, you have to advocate for yourself, but remember that doctors are used to being in control. All of the other patients come into the room with immediate respect, but your understanding has torn down the doctor–god illusion. That's a good thing in the long-run, but few doctors want to be greeted with that reality from the start. Your goal with any doctor is to build a partnership of trust that goes both ways, and coming on too strong at the start can hurt your chances of ever having that.

2.Show respect – I say this one carefully, because there are certainly some doctors who don't treat patients with respect – especially ones like you with chronic disease. These doctors should be avoided. But most of us are not like that; we really want to help people and try to treat them well. But we have worked very hard to earn our position; it was not bestowed by fiat or family tree. Just as you want to be listened to, so do we.

3.Keep your eggs in only a few baskets – find a good primary care doctor and a couple of specialists you trust. Don't expect a new doctor to figure things out quickly. It takes me years of repeated visits to really understand many of my chronic disease patients. The best care happens when a doctor understands the patient and the patient understands the doctor. This can only happen over time. Heck, I struggle even seeing the chronically sick patients for other doctors in my practice. There is something very powerful in having understanding built over time.

4.Use the ER only when absolutely needed – Emergency Room physicians will always struggle with you. Just expect that. Their job is to decide if you need to be hospitalized, if you need emergency treatment, or if you can go home. They might not fix your pain, and certainly won't try to fully understand you. That's not their job. They went into their specialty to fix problems quickly and move on, not manage chronic disease. The same goes for any doctor you see for a short time: they will try to get done with you as quickly as possible.

5.Don't avoid doctors – one of the most frustrating things for me is when a complicated patient comes in after a long absence with a huge list of problems they want me to address. I can't work that way, and I don't think many doctors can. Each visit should address only a few problems at a time, otherwise things get confused and more mistakes are made. It's OK to keep a list of your own problems so things don't get left out – I actually like getting those lists, as long as people don't expect me to handle all of the problems. It helps me to prioritize with them.

6.Don't put up with the jerks – unless you have no choice (in the ER, for example), you should keep looking until you find the right doctor(s) for you. Some docs are not cut out for chronic disease, while some of us like the long–term relationship. Don't feel you have to put up with docs who don't listen or minimize your problems. At the minimum, you should be able to find a doctor who doesn't totally suck.

7.Forgive us – Sometimes I forget about important things in my patients' lives. Sometimes I don't know you've had surgery or that your sister comes to see me as well. Sometimes I avoid people because I don't want to admit my limitations. Be patient with me – I usually know when I've messed up, and if you know me well I don't mind being reminded. Well, maybe I mind it a little.

You know better than anyone that we docs are just

people – with all the stupidity, inconsistency, and fallibility that goes with that – who happen to doctor for a living. I hope this helps, and I really hope you get the help you need. It does suck that you have your problem; I just hope this perhaps decreases that suckishness a little bit.

Sincerely,
Dr. Rob

APPENDIX I
POEM
(A POEM WRITTEN BY SOMEONE WITH RSD)

This poem was written by Darlene Brownell. Darlene is an RSD Patient. Thank you for Darlene for allowing me to share this with you.

Who Am I?

You can't see me, you can't hear me. I'm the one inside of you, making you go crazy. All the doctors you have seen, they still don't know me, that's funny to me. And it's been over 100 years. And they still can't find me, those tests they take and pictures, there just wasting there time. I told you before they won't find me no matter how hard they try. Indeed I'm the one that makes you hurt all day long. I am the one responsible for your terrible burning pain. I love burning you with my flames, keep complaining no one hears you, no one cares. They can't see me they cant feel me. I'm the only one who knows what you're feeling because your body belongs to me now, and I have the power to make your pain spread. So don't try to stop me, because you no what they will say, it's all in your head and how many pain meds have you taken today. Wow! There still saying that now, that's insane. I will leave you with nothing, no family and friends. I will keep torturing each and ever day till the bitter end because people can't see your pain and that makes my day. I'm going to take my flames and burn you in the worse possible way, I enjoy those shooting pains I give you threw out the day. HA– HA don't you wish you were dead, because that's my intent. If your doctor keeps giving you those meds it's going to affect you and mess with your head. That's ok he's doing my job, the more suffering you have makes me want to stay. I'm not leaving so stop praying; wipe your tears this nightmare is just beginning. Yes your really are a wake, I find that quite funny you thought it was a dream, It sucks to be you since no one understands. So do me a favor and do yourself in. Ok, I will tell you who and what I am. My name is called RSD isn't that a nice name. It stands for Rapid Spreading Disease. So tell that to all the morons you see. And maybe one day they will try and stop me. Bye the way would you please stop changing my name.

APPENDIX J
FIGHTING THE INSURANCE COMPANY: KETAMINE INFUSIONS

If you want your insurance company to cover Ketamine Infusions and they are telling you that they are either "experimental", "educational" or "investigational"; here's what you need to do. First you need the written denial. Most likely their reason for denying the treatment will be that it is experimental, or investigational.

You need to establish that you have CRPS/RSD by getting your RSD doctor to write a strong letter stating that you have severe RSD that will only respond to Ketamine.
You need to write a BRIEF history of your RSD experience.

For example here is mine:

*March of 1996 Franc Liss Fracture of right foot resulting in burning pain treated by casting and PT

*March of 1997 After a year of continued extreme pain, a fusion was done of right foot

*December of 1997, I was referred to an outpatient Chronic Pain Program at Bryn Mawr Rehabilitation Hospital when burning pain, purplish discoloration and swelling remained in the right foot. This program was run by a physiatrist and included PT, OT, individual psychology, group therapy and biofeedback. The Physiatrist ordered a three phase bone scan which showed that I most likely had RSD. He started me on Neurontin and referred me to Hahnemann's Neurology Clinic.

*April 1998, I saw Dr. (put your doctors name in)who did a Laser Doppler Study and Bier Block. She confirmed the diagnosis of RSD.

*1998 – 1999; multiple blocks including lumbar sympathetic, and thoracic. Pain spread up the right side and to the left side. Hospitalized for continuous epidurals,

*Lidocaine drips and finally for a trial of a medication pump.

*February 1999; Medtronic Medication Pump was placed. Increasing amounts of medication were needed to get any relief.

*2001; Dr. ___left the practice and care transferred to Dr. ___. who suggested Ketamine Coma Treatment in Germany in October.

*Feb 2002 – 2009 Ketamine out patient Ketamine infusions and inpatient awake infusions maintained my pain at a tolerable level.

(notice that I didn't go into the fact that I had my gallbladder out, had cancer, had back surgery, etc because it isn't relevant to my case for Ketamine)

You need to show them that Ketamine is no longer considered experimental. I have put together this set of paragraphs showing scientific studies that Ketamine is now considered Level I treatment for CRPS. PA Dept of Health review a case where Ketamine was denied and the appeals denied. I have the wording that got insurance to reverse their denial. Here it is.

There is nothing in the language of the health plan's Definition of Medical Necessity that would prevent the enrollee from continuing to look for further treatment options for refractory CRPS. IV Ketamine treatment is medically appropriate for the my condition/ It is given to improve physiological function; consistent with the current medical literature. It is consistent with the diagnosis of the condition; is not given for convenience; and not considered experimental for me per the current standards of care in the medical community.

In regard to the Ketamine infusion, if the health plan considers Ketamine therapy to be "Experimental or Investigational" treatment for of refractory CRPS then based on the discussion below, and the fact that non-anesthetic dose IV Ketamine is now supported by LEVEL I data in the literature, I feel that the I do meet the criteria to receive this form of treatment.

The health plan deemed the use of IV Ketamine to be not "Medically Necessary", but also stated that it was against the health plan's policy because it was considered "Experimental or Investigational". This is not an accurate statement and goes against the available medical literature. There are now two publications in the peer-reviewed literature that have LEVEL I date, derived from Phase III randomized, placebo-controlled clinical trials supporting the use of sub-anesthetic level IV Ketamine in patients with refractory CRPS Type 1 (6,7) In the study by Sigtermans et al, they studied sixty (60) patients and noted a statistically significant improvement in pain control (p<0.001) in the group of patients and noted a statistically significant improvement in pain control (p<0.001) in the group of patients receiving IV Ketamine in comparison to the group that received the placebo infusion. The study by Schwartzman et al was designed very similarly and also noted a statistically significant improvement in pain control (p<0.05) in the group receiving IV Ketamine. In an older paper by DR ME Goldberg you could support the position that IV Ketamine was experimental/investigational However, Dr Goldberg's position is further clarified in a more recent publication (8) In this paper, he does not state that IV Ketamine is not efficacious or appropriate for patients with severe or refractory CRS, nor does he state that it should be considered only an experimental or investigational treatment modality. What he does say is that there is selectivity in the responsiveness of various patients with CRPS to IV Ketamine and that this aspect of its use is still unclear and will require further study. Therefore, impatient admission for the admission of IV Ketamine is considered the standard of care in this enrollee's case.

References: These studies were printed out and sent in with the appeal. As you saw, they reviewer sited these studies when he reversed the insurance company's decision.

1. Brehl S. An update on the pathophysiology of complex regional pain syndrome. Anesthesiol 2010;113:713-725.

2. Albazaz R, Wong YT, Homer-Vanniasinkam S. Complex regional pain syndrome; a review. Ann Vasc Surg 2008;22:425-429.

3. Rowbotham MC. Pharmacologic management of complex regional pain syndrome. Clin J Pain 2006:22:425-429.

4. Ben-Ari A, Lewis MC, Davidson E. Chronic administration of Ketamine for analgesia. J Pan Palliat Care Pharmocother 2007;21:7-14.

5. Correll GE, Maleki J, Gracely EJ et al. Subanesthetic Ketamine infusion therapy; a retrospective analysis of a novel therapeutic approach to CRPS. Pain Med 2004:5:263-275.

6. Sigtermans MJ, van Hilten JJ, Bauer MC, et al. Ketamine produces effective and long-term pain relief in patients with complex regional pain syndrome type 1. Pain 2009;145:304-311.

7. Schwartzman RJ, Alexander GM, Grothusen JR, et al. Outpatient intravenous Ketamine for the treatment of complex regional pain syndrome; a double-blind placebo controlled study. Pain 209;147:107-115.

8. Goldberg ME, Schwartzman RJ, Torjman MC et al. Ketamine infusion successful in some patients. Pain Physician 2010; 13:E371-372.

(I suggest that you print them out & send them to your Insurance Co. The links are listed in Appendix G).

APPENDIX K
QUESTIONS TO ASK YOUR DOCTOR
When Interviewing Him/Her About Ketamine Treatments

Ask about their Ketamine Protocol:
Is pre-treatment testing needed? If so, what it is?
What is the Ketamine dosage?
Is the Ketamine given in patient or out patient?
Frequency of Infusions?
How do they handle IV access?
Who over sees the actual infusion?

Ask about the setting that the infusion is given in:

* Is it a private room or a group setting

*Are there beds/stretchers/recliners?

*Noise levels?

*May I bring my own pillow & blanket?

*May I bring my own music with head set?

*How long have they been administering Ketamine:

*What kind of lab work do they do before and after the infusions at what frequency?

*What happens if I need an infusion in between my regular infusions due to a fall or a major exacerbation?

*If you are coming from out of town; is there any discounted hotel arrangement available?

APPENDIX L
DOCUMENT TO GIVE TO HEALTHCARE WORKERS

HEALTHCARE WORKERS GUIDE TO CARING FOR THE CRPS/RSD PATIENT
By Nancy Renée Cotterman
© 2013

What the heck is CPRS/RSD?

This disease dates back to the Civil War. Soldiers who were wounded would complain of extreme pain. They would describe it as if a fire were burning on the affected limb. Doctors recognized it as a disease but they didn't quite know how to treat it or why it developed in some soldiers and not others with the exact type of wound. In that era doctors didn't share theories or treatments with each other, each one worked with their own patients trying different things to try to reduce their patient's pain.

Today doctors and researchers still aren't one hundred percent clear on what causes CPRS/RSD to develop in one person and not in another with the same type of injury. It is known by two main names; CRPS (Complex Regional Pain Syndrome) and RSD/RSDS (Reflex Sympathetic Pain Syndrome.)Many physicians and nurses still do not know what CRPS/RSD is so they do not know how to diagnose and treat these patients. Others have misconceptions about CRPS/RSD, such as: it can not spread, it doesn't cause widespread edema (swelling) and that the pain can not be debilitating. Many with CRPS/RSD are told that the pain is in their heads and not real. It is very real! It is important to treat the person with CRPS/RSD with dignity and respect as this is a very real and debilitating chronic pain disease.

So what exactly is RSD? It is a chronic neurological syndrome that is characterized by a severe burning pain that is often described by patients as if someone poured lighter fluid on them and then lit it or the most severe sunburn that you can have one thousand fold. They feel like they are on literally on fire. There are also pathological changes in the bone and the skin, such as bone loss, and shinny, hairless reddish purple skin. Many RSD patients have excessive sweating all of the time. The tissues of the effective area(s) swell. Most have an extreme sensitivity to touch (allodynia). Something as light as a breeze can cause excruciating pain. Clothing on the affecting area(s) can be painful. This last symptom can also cause people with RSD to pull away from the ones that they love as well as the hospital staff. Touch is a universal sign of friendship and love. Many people can't understand why the person is constantly pushing them away and asking them not to touch. Why? Because to someone with RSD, touch is extremely painful. Other stimuli such as bright light and noise can also be extremely painful to the person with CRPS/RSD/

Anyone can get RSD. It is more prevalent in women than men and the number of pediatric cases is on the rise. One of the biggest challenges that the RSD patient face is the lack of proper understanding and education of pain in the medical community. The inability to get insurance companies to recognize and pay for a multidisciplinary treatment team. Finally, the loss of employment, social structure and family life are all struggles that the patient with RSD may be faced with. One of the biggest battles is that of getting treatments covered by health insurance and workman's compensation insurance and access to the traditional medical routes. This forces them to often rely on emergency rooms for pain management.

RSD is a malfunction of part of the nervous system that usually develops in response to a traumatic even such as an accident or medical procedure. A minor injury such as a sprain or a fall can also cause nerves to misfire sending constant pain signals to the brain. These signals cause a memory within the nervous system which causes the patient to feel as though the injury has never healed. As time goes on, these pain signals become exaggerated and create a memory within the nervous system even after the original injury has healed.

CRPS/RSD is broken down into two categories:
CRPS I (RSD)
The symptoms of type I include: The presence of an imitating event such as a fracture, a crush injury, a splinter or sprain. Continuing pain including allodynia, which is pain from a normal stimulus such as the breeze from a ceiling fan, or hyperalgesia which an increased sense of pain. The pain is disproportionate to that associated with the injury. There is edema (swelling), changes in skin blood flow (skin color changes, skin temperature changes) and excessive sweating in the region of pain.

The diagnosis of CRPS I (RSD) is one of exclusion. It is based on the existence of conditions that would otherwise account for the degree of pain and dysfunction. There is no one diagnostic test that can show that CRPS/RSD is present.

CRPS II (Causalgia):
This is the presence of constant pain, allodynia (pain resulting from normal stimulus) or hyperalgesia (an increased sense of pain) after an identifiable nerve injury. Evidence of edema, and skin changes. This diagnosis is also one of exclusion based on the existence of conditions that would otherwise account for the degree of pain and dysfunction. The only difference between type I and type II is the actual nerve injury.

Tips on taking care of the CPRS/RSD Patient:

When making your initial assessment
Complex Regional Pain Syndrome (CRPS)/RSD is a chronic condition characterized by severe burning pain, pathological changes in bone and skin, excessive sweating, tissue swelling and extreme sensitivity to touch, light and noise. People afflicted with RSD/CRPS are extraordinarily sensitive to certain stimuli, such as touch, movement, bright light, noise and injections.

*Always ask the patient before touching them!

*Ask the person about their CPRS/RSD;
Where is their pain exactly?

*Are their things that make it worse? Better?

*Have them rate their pain level for you.

*When taking BP, ask which extremity they would prefer it being taken on. Manual BP cuffs are less painful than automatic ones and should be used when available. Use thigh cuff if both upper extremities are affected

*Any breeze, sheet, blanket can cause an increase in pain, inquire before covering any part of the body to be sure that it won't increase their pain.

*Ask what temperature is best for them (some people don't tolerate heat and others don't tolerate cold).

*If possible, place a sign above bed designating affected limb(s).

IVs and Blood work:
Any venapuncture can cause extreme pain for the person with CRPS/RSD. It can be a cause of spread of the disease. Use pediatric needles (any trauma can cause the spread of CRPS to a new site) and pediatric blood tubes for collecting blood samples. Ask the patient if there are any areas that should not be used for an IV or blood draw.

Never tap on the vein to bring it up as this can cause extreme pain and often causes the veins of a CPRS/RSD patient to disappear.

Warm the area of blood draw or IV stick. CRPS/RSD patients often are hard sticks.

Warm alcohol or betadine wipes with warm running water on outside of package before opening package (these wipes can be very cold to the patient).

Warming IV medications prior to infusion can decrease the pain and inflammation to the veins.

If PICC site is available, see if blood can be obtained from PICC instead of using venapuncture technique.

Dos and Don'ts for the care of the CRPS/RSD patient:
CRPS/RSD is a chronic pain syndrome that varies from person to person in the exact symptoms. The main symptom is constant burning pain that is exacerbated by touch, movement, light, noise and temperature.

Ask before touching the patient.

Avoid using ice. This can cause spread of the CRPS/RSD.

Often having their own pillows, sheets and blankets from home can make the patient tolerate their hospital environment better as hospital sheets, blankets and pillows can be irritating to the patient.

Bright light and loud noise can be extremely painful to the person with CRPS/RSD as the patients are extremely sensitive to these stimuli. Turning off fluorescent lights and minimizing extraneous noise can help to make the patient more comfortable whenever possible.

In transferring the patient: Ask what kind of help the patient needs when transferring to a stretcher or wheelchair (simply touching arms or legs may cause hyperalgesia). Use extreme care over bumps, such as elevator doorways.

Please place all hospital bracelets on an unaffected limb. The addition of a red bracelet to designate that the patient has CPRS/RSD and place red dot sticker on patient chart or write in red on the patient chart can signal to other staff members that the patient has CRPS/RSD.

The main thing in caring for a patient with CRPS/RSD is

to be sure to ask before touching the patient and be as knowledgable about the disease as possible. Some great resources are:

www.RSDSA.org
www.RSDHope.org
www.crpapartnersinpain.com

APPENDIX M
MY EMERGENCY KIT

In a zippered case like this one to the right, I keep copies of important papers that are accessible to everyone in the family in case of an emergency. This case Includes:

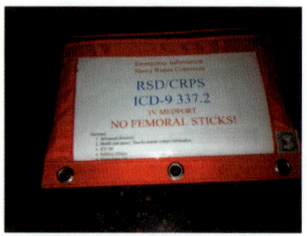

* My advanced directive

  *A summary of my medical history

* An up to date copy of my medication list including my allergies as well as the name and phone number of my pharmacy

* A list of all of my treating physicians with their names, addresses, phone number, and specialty

 *RSD for health care providers sheet

  *A kit to access my port

APPENDIX N
IV ACCESS

When you have made the decision to get IV Ketamine or Lidocaine you need to make an educated decision as to how the medications should be infused into your body. This decision needs to be made in conjunction with your doctor.

For the most part, when you enter into treatment with Ketamine/Lidocaine for RSD, it is an ongoing treatment if it is successful. This should be taken into consideration when deciding what type of IV access you want.

If your first Ketamine/Lidocaine treatment is outpatient and you are not sure how it will work for you; as Ketamine/Lidocaine is not always the best treatment for everyone, then a traditional peripheral IV may be your best access. The peripheral IV must be changed every 72 hours (in most facilities). When you are getting outpatient treatments, most facilities will allow you to go home with the IV in place for three days of outpatient infusions. They will take steps to protect the catheter when you are at home so that it doesn't get dislodged. There is always the chance that it will become dislodged and wil need to be replaced. Lidocaine or EMLA cream (numbing medications) can be used when a peripheral IV is started. There have been some cases where the placement of an IV has caused spread of RSD. I could not find any percentages of cases where the spread of RSD was associated with an IV stick. Here is what a peripheral IV looks like:

Source of photo:
http://en.wikipedia.org/wiki/
File:Intravenous_therapy_2007-SEP-13-Singapore.JPG

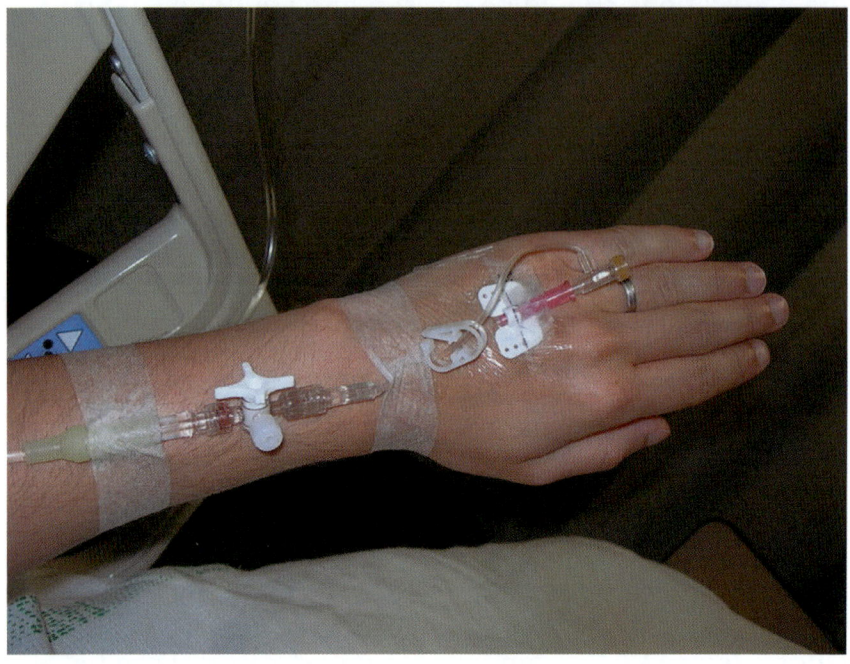

If your first Ketamine/Lidocaine treatment is inpatient; you will most likely be getting follow up "booster" infusions. In this case, it makes more sense that you get a more permanent access. One form of permanent IV access is a mediport/portacath. This is surgically implanted, usually in your chest just under the skin, and is accessed by a special needle called a Huber needle. The surgeon could use removable sutures or dissolvable sutures. You should inquire which the surgeon is using because this makes a difference in your recovery. For the non-RSD patient, the removal of sutures is normally painless. As a RN, I've taken them out hundreds of times and my patients have never complained. For the RSD patient, the removal of sutures can be painful because we are more sensitive. Dissolvable sutures with steri-strips can be used in the placement of a port. It is the surgeon's choice. You, as the consumer, need to know which your doctor prefers to use and discuss it with the physician.

When the port is not being used, there is just a slight bulge under the skin. When it is being used, the Huber needle is inserted through the skin and into a reservoir just under the skin and secured with a clear dressing. The Huber needle can stay in place for up to seven days. After the 7 days, the needle must be changed if IV access is still needed. The risk of infection is very low with this type of device. The port is accessed under sterile conditions. It does require monthly flushing by a nurse to keep it patent. This can be done in your doctor's office.

Here is some information on the mediport/portacath:

Source of photo: http://en.wikipedia.org/wiki/Port_(medical)
This is what the port looks like before

Some This is what the looks like when not accessed. This is what it looks like when accessed.

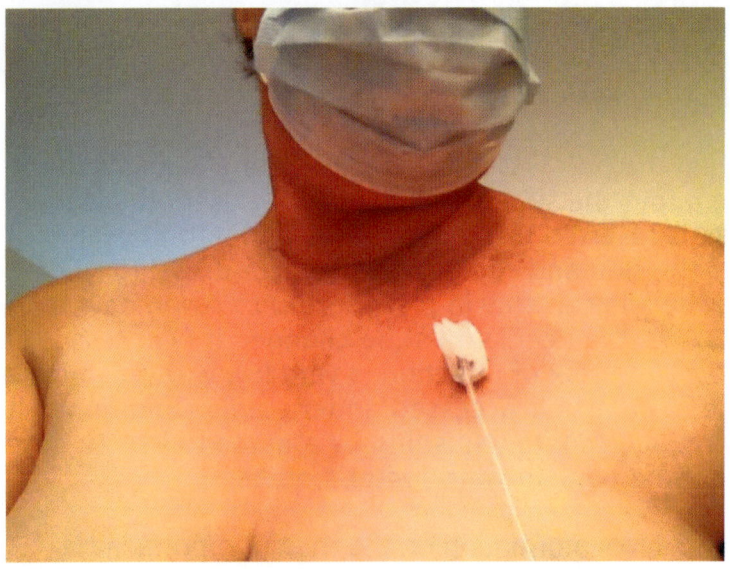

An
accessed port

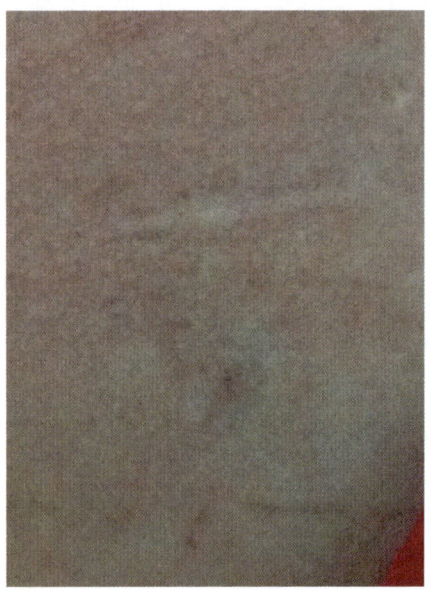

An healed port not accessed

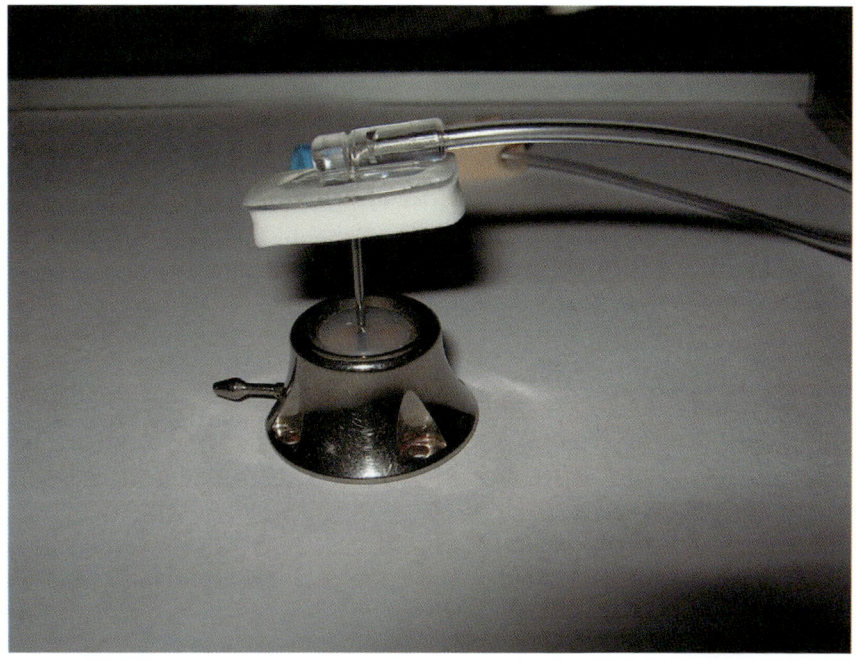

The actual equipment placed inside the chest and accessed with a huber needle.

Benefits of the Mediport/Portacath System Include:
It minimizes damage to veins, muscle and skin tissue by allowing the medication to be diluted faster in the larger veins

It allows for a single location that your doctor can use to infuse medications or take blood directly from large veins.

It avoids the risk and pain to the RSD patient of looking for new veins each time the patient needs an infusion or have a blood sample taken.

Scar tissue builds up over time at the Mediport/Portacath location making each needle penetration less painful over time.

Minimizes risk of infection over a temporary central line. Can be left in place for years with proper maintenance (monthly flushing)

There are other central line options that include a PICC line (peripherally inserted central line) which usually is place into the arm. On the outside, it looks like a regular IV but the catheter is longer and goes into a larger vein.

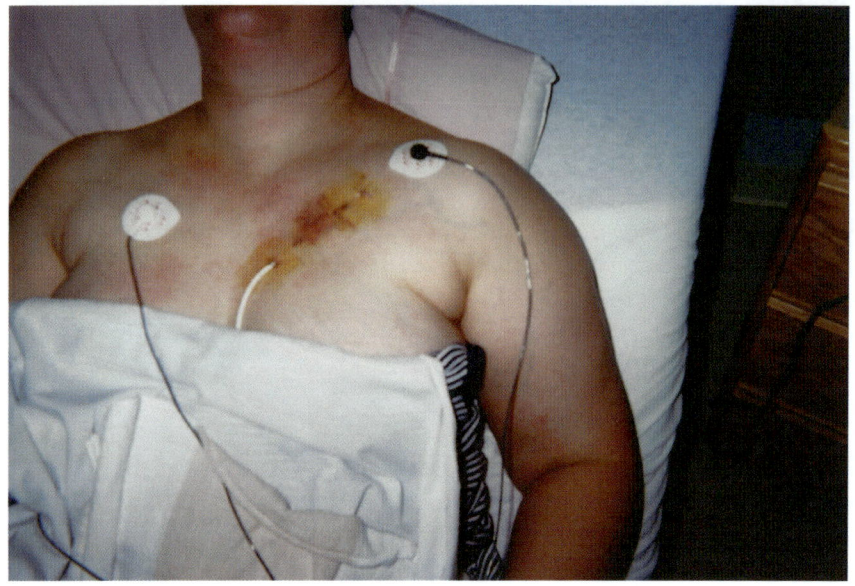

This is a Hickman Catheter newly placed.

The Hickman, and a non–tunneled central lines; which are placed in the chest area.

There are central lines that are just sutured into place that can be put into the jugular vein in the neck or the femoral vein in the groin. There are other central lines, but these are the most common. Here is a Wikipedia explanation of some types of central lines. Most of these types of central lines are temporary in nature and are removed before you are discharged from the hospital. The

Mediport/portacath   and Hickman can be left in place for years.

http://en.wikipedia.org/wiki/Central_venous_catheter

As you can see, if you are going into the hospital for inpatient IV therapy, how the medication is going to be infused is something that you need to think about and discuss with your physician BEFORE you are admitted. You don't want to find out the morning of admission that you are getting a different type of IV access than you thought or that you are getting removable sutures rather than dissolvable sutures and steri-strips. You don't want to find out upon discharge when you are sleepy and possibly still disoriented that your IV access is being removed; when you thought that it was staying in place for future infusions. This is just another part of your informed decision that you need to make when planning your RSD treatment.

APPENDIX O
RSD AND MEMORY

RSD PUZZLE # 107

Poor Memory And Visual Problems: RSD Has Four Principles

1. Hyperpathic and allodynic pain

2. Muscle contraction in vessel walls and in extremities

3. Inflammation (edema, ulcers, etc...)

4. The 4th principle is constant input of pain in the limbic system (Frontal and Temporal lobes) causing poor memory, irritability, insomnia, and agitation. Antidepressants, especially Trazodone or Desipramine and better control of pain, improve these complications. Another cause of poor memory is tendency for poor cerebral circulation.

Blurred vision, dizziness, and poor balance are common manifestations of RSD. The disease causes constriction of vertebral arteries resulting in poor circulation to the brain stem, this in turn causes poor focusing of eye muscles, and poor balance and dizziness. Proper cervical, paravertebral and epidural blocks correct these symptoms.

H. Hooshmand, M.D.

APPENDIX P
PRESCRIPTION DRUG PROGRAMS

There are programs that help people on a fixed income get free prescriptions or prescriptions at a reduced cost. Since most of us are on fixed incomes, I thought that this would be a relevant topic to post about. Here are some links:

http://www.medicationoutreach.com/site/

http://www.pparx.org/

http://www.rxassist.org/

http://www.medicare.gov/pharmaceutical-assistance-program/index.aspx?AspxAutoDetectCookieSupport=1

http://www.ncsl.org/issues-research/health/state-pharmaceutical-assistance-programs.aspx

5636222R00139

Printed in Great Britain
by Amazon.co.uk, Ltd.,
Marston Gate.